L.A.
from A to Z

THE
ACTOR'S GUIDE TO
Surviving and Succeeding
IN
LOS ANGELES

Thomas Mills

HEINEMANN, PORTSMOUTH, NH

For my wife, Wendy,
and
My mother, Maude

Two incredible forces in my life

Heinemann
A division of Reed Elsevier Inc.
361 Hanover Street
Portsmouth, NH 03801–3912
www.heinemanndrama.com

Offices and agents throughout the world

© 2002 by Thomas Mills

Library of Congress Cataloging-in-Publication Data
Mills, Thomas, 1959–
    LA from A to Z : the actor's guide to surviving and succeeding in
Los Angeles / Thomas Mills.
        p. cm.
    ISBN 0-325-00397-1
    1. Acting—Vocational guidance—California—Los Angeles.   I. Title.
PN2055 .M55 2002
792′.028′02379494—dc21   2002027617

Editor: Lisa A. Barnett
Production service: TechBooks
Production coordinator: Sonja S. Chapman
Cover design: Linda Knowles
Manufacturing: Steve Bernier
Compositor: TechBooks

Printed in the United States of America on acid-free paper
06 05 04 03 02 VP 1 2 3 4 5

Contents

E

F

G

H

I

J

K

L

M

N

O

P

Q

R

S

T

U

V

W

X, Y, & Z

Acknowledgments

I've always thought the acknowledgments section was a bit of a pressure cooker for an author. I mean, honestly, who do you thank? If I had to put together an accurate list of those who have helped me through the years—and ultimately in my journey as a person who happens to be an actor who happens to be writing a book about being an actor—well, it would be a lot longer than this sentence.

So before mentioning just a few specific names, I'll do a universal recognition of my sincerest gratitude to everyone I know, have known, and hope to know someday . . . just in case I've left you off the list.

First and foremost, beyond any level that I could express in words, is my love and respect for my wife, Wendy. Her companionship, support, and love deserve a volume of books of their very own.

I've known so many actors through the years who became great friends, and I'll mention just a few here: Glenn Michael Herrera, Paul Hartel, Gretchen Koerner, Joey Perillo, Dominick "Foo" Lucente, James Hassett, Erik St. Anthony, and Oscar Torres. Some are quoted in the book, and others have shared their industry stories and thoughts with me throughout the years. Much of what they've expressed to me is represented in these pages.

I've been writing the "Tombudsman" column for *Backstage West* newspaper for eight years now. That blows me away, that I've done anything for eight years, but so I have. I've had literally thousands of actors write me—of which many have never had their questions answered in the paper. There's only so much space in a column. I thank them for their loyalty and only wish I was able to answer all the questions that you've posted to me. To those of you to whom I have been able to respond, I thank you for sharing your stories and adventures, your sorrows and triumphs. They have educated and comforted many of your fellow performers, and helped get me to the point where I am able to actually attempt a book.

I'd also like to thank Editor in Chief and Associate Publisher at *Backstage West*, Rob Kendt, for listening to me all those years ago when I pitched an idea for a serious Q&A column, "Tombudsman," and my thespian-on-the-street monthly essay, "Working Actor." Thankfully, he went for both. I'd also like to salute the staff, present and past, at the paper for all their help throughout the years—Jim, those carica-tures make that one Thursday a month worth waiting for. I'm in-debted to Managing Editor Scott Proudfit for his support each and every week.

The other editor in my life, Lisa Barnett at Heinemann, has been the best. Not only did she approach me about writing for her company—that's a dream for a writer—but she has given me free reign to write the book I wanted to write. Her sense of humor and flexible definition of "due date" were much appreciated by the first-time book writer. And to the entire crew at Heinemann and TechBooks, my deepest appreciation for all of your efforts put forth in completing the project.

I have been fortunate enough to be a working actor now and again, and have met and worked alongside an incredible amount of wonderful people on both sides of the camera in Los Angeles. Many have left an indelible impression on me, including James Brolin, Ken Olin, Hart Bochner, Mel Smith, Jill Hennessey, Dennis Franz, Alan Rosenberg, Stephen Rea, Michael Moriarity, and the late Elizabeth Montgomery, who I was privileged to work with on her last film. What do all these people have in common, aside from being exemplary in their work? They are all class acts, wonderful, respectful individuals. A perfect work day to me is not just acting—it's being on the set with people who have a high regard and respect for one another. That's what all these people have in common. You'll work with many people in your career and be blessed to share time with folks like those I've mentioned.

A special thanks to Karen Kondazian, a wonderful actress and writer who was always there to lend me a kind word and a helpful tip about this book writing business.

I'd also like to acknowledge actress and coach Daphne Eckler Kirby for her contribution, assistance, and ever-present good cheer, and for being my first acting teacher when I came to Los Angeles. I'm still using what you taught me, Daphne.

During the preparation for this book, I spoke with casting directors, agents, actors, managers, instructors, and other entertainment profes-sionals. All shared their industry perspective with me, and many are quoted in these pages. I thank them for their generosity of time and for their insights on the acting industry.

My gratitude also to the staff at Starbucks at the Howard Hughes Center and Anastasia's in Santa Monica where I did so much of this writing wired up on caffeine. Thanks for the java, the work space, and for not charging me rent. You certainly had every right to.

David Rosenbaum, a long-time friend from New York City, has been a continuing source of encouragement for me throughout the years and is one of those great people who every year assures me the big one is coming. I always hope he doesn't mean an earthquake.

Finally, but certainly not least, I thank my family. They are an eclectic and diverse bunch, spread out from New Jersey, to New York, to Connecticut, to Washington, DC, to Florida, to Studio City. I love you all. Send pictures, please. And to you, this book's reader, whether new to the industry and city, or seasoned performer, I hope you find great happiness and success in this dynamic field.

Introduction—What This Book Is and Isn't . . .

The shelves of any Los Angeles bookstore are overflowing with a ton of titles about making it as an actor in film and television. Some offer practical advice from knowledgeable sources and some are written by people who wouldn't know a close-up from a craft services table. Most of them, whether valid or not, are trying to help actors find the key to unlock the door to Hollywood success.

I don't want to waste your time. This isn't that kind of book. I certainly want to help you succeed, but I just don't have that key. In fact, I don't subscribe to this whole key to success theory, nor do I buy into the *making it* mentality.

The acting field is as wide open a profession as there ever was. There is no "one" way to make it—no hard and fast rules to follow that'll guarantee you any degree of success. Two actors could follow the exact same career plan, right down to the teachers, the auditions, and the style of headshots, and yet end up at opposite ends of the success chart. There are so many variables, tangible and otherwise.

Besides, the whole concept of making it is one that professional actors know is as much a fiction as what Hollywood puts up on the big screen. Actors don't make it or not make it. That's tourist talk. What's making it anyway, doing a couple of dayplayer jobs per year, having your own television series, bringing in one million dollars per year, two million dollars, perhaps? Is there some chart on a wall that says this gig plus that paycheck equals success?

No way. Success for a professional actor comes down to one thing—commitment. How far he goes with his work in the public eye, or as measured by his paycheck, is something for others to ponder.

Whether hitting the stage in a ninety-nine-seat theatre on Santa Monica Boulevard or showing up at a Universal sound stage to play a cop in a sitcom, LA actors act, try to act some more, and that's that. They go through their careers repeating that on again–off again cycle, and maybe they eventually land a big gig and someone declares, "See, they made it."

No. They'd made it all along, just by surviving as an actor. So I don't believe in or care to write about making it, but I do get excited when discussing actor survival. That's a subject I can really get into.

In surviving, if you manage to make a living at what you love, then no matter where you end up on the great wall of acting, you are a success.

Surviving is that time between jobs, and sometimes even during jobs, when you are living your career. It's has its ups, its way ups, its downs, its way downs, and its lots of in-betweens (*waiting,* in acting parlance), and it's always a challenge.

I've been fortunate to survive for nearly twenty years as an actor—eight of them here in Los Angeles—and have paid my dues, paid them again, and will probably continue to pay them. I've had great years, and less than stellar ones. That's an actor's life. A plumber needs a wrench to do his job, a doctor a stethoscope, whereas actors need the acceptance of unknowing. That's a legitimate job tool. Similar to any professional performer, I'm thrilled when I get a job, but I also realize that a week later I'll probably be unemployed again. The survival cycle kicks in anew.

You know what? Most actors will tell you, that's just fine. After all, we are privileged to do what we do, even if we spend much of our time trying to get work rather than actually doing it. Though we don't define success by the size of the residual check, amount of attendees in the orchestra section, or how many people recognize us in the shopping mall, we like to work. Hopefully, the words on these pages will help to get your momentum moving more in that employment direction.

The A–Z topics in this book serve as a highlight reel on many of the important areas you'll face as an actor in Los Angeles. There are nearly a hundred categories and several subcategories written about—some short, some extensive—and you'll eventually encounter most of them while living and working in LA.

By placing the categories alphabetically, I'm hoping you'll get more practical use from the book over time as a reference source. There were certainly no shortage of subjects to consider including in the book. I eventually selected the topics that I felt would be most beneficial to both the neophyte and the experienced actor. I believe I've picked many of the issues that have the most relevance on a day-to-day basis for working-class actors who are of this beautiful city. You'll find the industry categories you would expect, such as *agents, casting directors,* and *marketing.* You'll also see material that isn't in most of the other books but is nearly as important to an actor's daily life as having a great headshot. I'll cover things like *self-esteem,* head games in the *waiting room,* and those *zero audition* phases. These are issues that actors face all the time but yet are rarely written about.

I'll also touch on a few nonindustry elements of living in this city that sometimes affect what happens to you as an actor—like two of LA's premiere topics of conversation—*traffic* and *earthquakes.*

I've worked to put together a collection of material that is serious and fun, pragmatic and honest. I think the combination of those four ingredients is also a healthy approach to being an actor.

This book is both subjective, based on what I've personally learned and experienced as an actor in Los Angeles, and objective in that it also encapsulates the stories and themes of the hundreds of actors I've been in contact with during the past eight years that I've written the "Tombudsman" column for *Backstage West.* Aside from my personal recollections, if it's covered here, you can be assured I've heard it echoed time and time again from other actors as well. Then there are the casting directors, agents, managers, directors, and producers I've worked with and learned from. Their words of wisdom about the industry are reflected in these pages, sometimes in quote and other times in spirit.

Throughout the book, I will refer to the *average actor.* This is not a reflection of someone's talent. Most of us are in fact the average actor. By average, I mean someone who is talented and employable, but not a star; marketable, but not a ringer; working, but never enough. That's the average actor in Los Angeles, and it's also the majority. Until you land a series with your name in the title or a lead in a blockbuster film, you are also part of that fold.

You won't find the key to success here because there isn't one key that fits the Hollywood door. There are many that unlock various doors, and they come in a multitude of shapes and sizes—no two actors open them the same way. But even if there isn't "a way" to make it in Hollywood, I know there are certainly methods, preferences, and common approaches that have worked for many before you. You'll discover some of them in here, and you might pick and choose the ones that suit you best and use them in your game plan.

Of course, everyone's acting journey in Los Angeles is unique, so this guide isn't meant to give you all the answers; it's more suggestive of scenarios you're likely to come across as a performer in LA. Then again, you may decide you have a better idea. As an actor, you are your own boss and can do that. The truth is, your way might be better. If it is, write a book and share it with us will you? Out there, doing it is where you find the real answers, in your own way and in your own time. This book will merely attempt to help you to focus on the realities of the acting scene as I and others have witnessed it.

Throughout these A–Zs, I'll focus on what I know—climbing the ladder, and it's rarely straight upward, and surviving through it all while building your way to a fulfilling and, hopefully, very long career in the acting industry.

Chapter One

Surviving To Succeed

Surviving as an actor in Los Angeles—sounds a little dramatic, huh? Perhaps, but right out of the gate you'd be smart to adopt that very mentality about this show business of Hollywood. Survival isn't just an option, it's a necessity if you hope to have any semblance of an ongoing career.

Ongoing, because that's what separates the nonsurvivors—many of whom might be terrific actors—from those who manage to combine ability with tenacity to succeed year after year in America's largest acting market.

They are true survivors and, if you're very fortunate, you'll be able to count yourself among the ranks. The fact is, unless you achieve superstardom, and that only happens to a few of the thousands who make their livings at this, actual acting will only be a part-time aspect of your career. If you talk to any working actor in Hollywood, they'll tell you that surviving between jobs is the real challenge. Surviving is your full-time job.

It's tough, but the good news is that it can be done. Many do it every day. Then again, just as many, if not more, roll up the tent and move on to more sensible careers. There's no shame in that, and a lot of people would admit it's downright smart to do so. However, if you absolutely refuse to leave this profession, this vocation, this quixotic blend of art and business, then you already have the survival instincts that are as necessary for acting success as a good 8×10.

The first key to survival is to understand what *real* acting success is. It's not just having a television series written for you, or having your name bandied about in the press for setting a new box office record—though these are certainly things that many hope to see one day. The true success story in Hollywood is an actor, at any level of his career, who works.

1

When you come to Hollywood and see firsthand that there are thousands of qualified and usually unemployed actors trying to do just that—get a day's work—you begin to realize the enormity of the situation. Whatever acting market you came from, surely you faced challenges, but this is something altogether different. There's a ton of work here during the busier seasons, particularly in the fall and spring, but there's also something else—actors, tons of them.

Two very important words to know in Hollywood are *supply* and *demand*. The supply is us and it's always ample; the demand is the amount of actual jobs to go around. You probably won't be shocked to hear that the latter is a much, much smaller number. What you do about it, how long and how well you do it, and whether you stick it out or head home to do theatre will ultimately define your Los Angeles experience.

Remember that you are entering a business that demands that you not only have talent, but also are smart enough to know what to do with it. Working actors are smart actors and although you'll occasionally discover someone with enormous success who has the intelligence of an avocado, you'll almost always be competing for work with people that would be enormously successful in any other career. They've just so happened to choose one of the toughest in the world in which to make their living.

It's not enough to just be a good actor. Good acting is a given. Among other qualities, you have to be talented, a solid and persistent marketer, a good communicator and team player, a financial magician (how else can you survive in a field where you might make $50,000 one year and $5000 the next), and a quick study, and you must have a bit of luck on your side, too. Although you are only a human full of fragility and questions, you need an unflappable strong belief in yourself. If you have that you're going to stand a much better chance of having others believe in you, too. That's when they hire you.

I am not going to pull any punches here, your chances of doing well are dramatically increased if you are young and beautiful. This is Hollywood after all. Now with that said, I will reassure those of you, and myself, who don't look anything like Tom Cruise or Charlize Theron that you can pretty much have *any* look and find success. It just won't be as easy but, as any professional can attest, when has acting ever been easy? Finding and maintaining success in our profession is flatout hard for everyone. Multiply that by about ten and you are beginning to understand what's going on in Los Angeles.

Do you accept that? Rather than fret about it, are you already determining a way to work within that framework? I'm here to tell you that it can be done. There is always room for another survivor in Hollywood.

Chapter Two

Career Acting

Let me tell you right away that I love acting, love it, at least the acting part anyway. Hollywood's a great city when you're working. Unfortunately, actual acting, and maybe even being paid well for it, encompasses only a small percentage of the overall time you'll devote to being a professional. The real job of being an actor means that you're in near-constant pursuit of applying for jobs. Huh? Exactly. If you're anything like the vast majority of actors, you'll be seeking work much more of the time than you'll actually be performing. That's survival at its core. Learn to accept and deal with that reality, and you'll be a long way ahead of the field.

Most of the time, working actors are out of work, although they're perpetually seeking it. And they're the successful ones! Frankly, most people who try to succeed in the acting field don't work at all or soon find a career that, even if it drives them nuts, at least includes a weekly check, a 401(K), and two weeks' paid vacation per year. Can you imagine a businessman getting a great position only to find out twenty-four hours later that his reward for a great first day on the job is that he's now unemployed again? So he goes out and applies for twenty-five other jobs, finally gets another, and is again out of work only a few days later, and on and on. Actors understand it all too well.

If you are able to survive the LA odds and find an acting job or two, you have succeeded in finding a job or two, but let's be honest, that's not a career. A career takes time and years of dedication, but you'd be amazed at the amount of people who come here and think that once they get that first job they are set for life. It just doesn't work that way.

No one expects an actor to go to a film set every day, but you've got to get there with some degree of regularity to have a fighting chance of a continuing career. Sooner or later, you have to come to terms with being both an artist and a professional actor. You've got to be good at your craft while also making a living at it, so you can pay the bills, have a decent place to live, and keep your car running.

LA is a tough place to do that, and it's almost impossible if you come unprepared. First, don't rush your arrival to the city. The image of a giddy newcomer making it big might still persist, but most neophytes without training, regional credits, and a resume that states "I am a professional" will not last long. Nearly every person who is supposedly discovered or plucked from obscurity has a true history that reveals years of training, performing, and paying their dues. Of course, there is that rare exception who flies into town without a clue and lands a series. The odds of this are about the same as getting hit by lightening—twice.

There are a lot of places where you can start as an actor, but if you're going to attempt it in LA you're going to have an extraordinary uphill battle. Get some experience elsewhere, build a starter resume at the very least, and only then consider coming here. Despite its laid-back reputation, LA is an intense place full of people who are all trying to survive in their own fashion.

Most *working* actors in Hollywood make their livings as journey-men players, hired as costars and guest stars for television and playing supporting roles in films. The occasional commercial comes along, and there are always the famous ninety-nine-seat Equity waiver houses, which, although giving you a chance to feel like a real actor, barely pay your transportation costs. There is also voice-over work, extra and stand-in gigs, industrials (but not many considering the market size), music videos, and a few larger Equity houses that offer substantial contracts. Collectively, there is a ton of work in Los Angeles, even though Canada has snatched a lot of it away, but there is never enough to go around. It's survival of the fittest, and patience is more than a virtue.

Yet, there are certainly worse places in the world to try to make a career. America's second largest city is an agreeable mix of commerce, culture, and natural beauty. Like every city, it has its problems—crime, homelessness, and trying to overcome the image of a long-embattled police department. Still, LA practically overflows with the energy born of a place that views itself as redefining what a twenty-first-century urban metropolis could be. Whatever it fully evolves into, one thing is for sure, it will remain the celluloid capital of the world.

Los Angeles and the film and television business are inseparable. At the cafe you love, they're doing a tech scout. Driving along the beach, you pull up to a stoplight and see a primetime star fixing a tire on his bike. Passing through downtown after midnight, there are not one or two but three active shoots going on within a block of each other. In one minimall in the Valley where you stop for coffee, there is a voice studio, an acting teacher's classroom, an on-camera workshop, and a headshot photographer. Your landlord in Toluca Lake is an actor/screenwriter and the building alone could support an independent film production—producer and actress on floor one, cinematographer and set designer on two, animator on three, and assistant director next door (that was my old building, by the way). On every third or fourth light pole, there's either a neon sign pointing you to another film set or an "Extras Wanted" flyer pasted by some questionable company. Circulating by the thousands at all points in the city are others such as yourself, actors seeking to get their piece of the pie.

If you succeed, you'll certainly have your good days and your triumphs. However, if your *working* career is anything like that of the multitude of others who have come west before you, you'll also hit the inevitable downtime and struggles that are an all-too-common reality of being a professional performer in a big city where there is too little work to go around.

That's when you really become a surviving actor. It's when things don't go well and seem to be getting worse, when despite all the odds, you look at yourself in the mirror and commit to sticking it out, even at the expense of things most people, who have a choice, would never think of doing without.

Career actors don't do this for the money, the fame, or the trailer they let you hang out in when you have a gig, they do it because they love the craft, the process, and most important, the 5:00 AM burrito, licorice, M&Ms, barley soup, Altoids snack combo.

You'll understand once you're on the set.

A

Acting Classes

LA offers actors every imaginable class, seminar, workshop, and study environment that you would expect in a city whose claim to fame is show business. There are literally hundreds of teachers, schools, and programs offered.

You'll have almost too many choices when it comes to making your decisions on where to study and to whom you're going to shell out your hard earned, and often limited, cash in the pursuit of being a better and hopefully gainfully employed performer.

You can study everything from Shakespeare to Stanislavsky, from Movement to Meisner, and from classical to contemporary, but it won't take you long in Los Angeles before you'll realize that by far the largest and most practical segment of acting instruction here is focused on what this metropolis is famous for—the film and television industry.

With all due respect to the rapidly growing reputation that the LA theatre has recently garnered, if you are like most actors who come to LA, you've primarily done so in pursuit of work on the small and big screen. Therefore, your frontline education must serve to help you increase your chances to land work in those mediums.

On-camera classes are the most sensible approach for an actor new to this market. Within the on-camera category are a wide variety of styles and specialties, including the two most popular, scene study and cold reading. Take all of the classes you need and can afford, just make sure one of them has a camera in the room.

If you've previously worked only on stage and aren't familiar with how you appear when being videotaped, you could be in for a big surprise. Aside from the common "bring it down" note that refugees from the stage get when they first appear on-camera, when you see yourself acting on tape or film, especially in close-up, you become aware of a whole new you. Do I really do that with my nose? Why are my hands waving around like a flag? What the hell am I looking at? You need to learn about this stuff in class, not on the day you get hired for a job on a multimillion-dollar film set.

Los Angeles acting teacher, Daphne Eckler Kirby, keys in on some training elements that are essential to helping you to become and stay a working actor in Hollywood:

> As most of the work here is in film and television, it's very valuable to be studying on-camera, and the script work is the whole enchilada here. You're auditioning with scripts and making specific choices from them. Knowing how to work in a particular genre, from all the different styles we have out here, sitcoms to sci-fi is also important. I have noticed that a lot of actors, however gifted, talented, and instinctual they may be are not focusing enough on the craft aspect. I think if you do, when things come up like nerves or intense competition, that each actor faces here going up for a role, the craft will get you through that.

The vast majority of teachers and acting schools offer some type of on-camera class or workshop, but your primary goal must be in finding the best instructor who also has her finger on the pulse of the industry. Acting skill is of utmost importance, but you cannot forget this is a business. A connected instructor can teach you as much about the business side as the craft.

Newcomer to Los Angeles, Michele Mirkin explains that that was part of her objective in choosing a teacher. "I was looking for someone who would be supportive but also realistic. What appealed to me about my teacher was that she also helps with your marketing."

How do you find a teacher? Books such as *The Working Actor's Directory* list many classes around Los Angeles. This is a good starting point, but ads and descriptions, although helpful, are no substitute for getting out on the street and doing your own deeper investigation.

Start by asking your fellow performers about their favorite acting teachers. More often than not, they are the ones with whom they are now studying. Compile a list of names and look for repeats. It's a big city with a lot of instructors, but you'll hear many of the same names repeatedly. When you've identified four or five candidates, then it's time to set up some appointments.

Most LA acting teachers will allow you to audit one class. This means you can sit in and watch as the teacher works with her students. It likely won't take more than a single class for you to know if the teacher's style connects for you and whether you want to commit to signing up for the class yourself. Auditing is a real privilege. As a passive observer, you can learn a lot and that's a class all by itself. You will not be allowed to participate in any way while auditing a class. The teacher will generally introduce the auditors to the class members, who have previously told the teacher it's okay to have viewers in class, and you'll smile, sit back, and take it all in.

Take note of the teacher's style, that is, how she relates to her students. I always put a lot of emphasis on feedback. One teacher I had gave such incredible feedback in the first five minutes of the class that I mentally signed up before the second scene was completed.

Also, pay attention to class size. Do the actors get ample time to perform? Nothing is worse than an overcrowded class where you find yourself a paying viewer rather than a paying actor.

Study the students themselves. Are they professional, supportive, and most important, do they seem motivated and prepared? Students who are unprepared with scenes, seem closed off from the teacher, or are confrontational when given feedback are usually indicative of a class on which you want to pass. Of course, you could just be there on a bad night, so if you still have interest you might want to ask for a second audit. The most the teacher can say is "no."

Although you don't want to judge anyone, you have every right to evaluate the acting in front of you. If the level is well below or even well above where you currently are in your own journey, you might need another class or another teacher. My goal for class has always been to be with actors I felt on par with or who were up a level from me. This helps you to grow professionally.

A teacher might suggest that you sign up for a beginning-level class when you think you're past that level. Let your ego down for a minute, hear him out, and you might find that the starting class is more advanced than you knew. If you have doubts, you can audit that particular class before committing.

If you're happy with what you've seen, then you might sign up as a student. Let's say it's a scene study class, on-camera, of course. You should consider that it's probably going to take a while before you get maximum benefit from the class. As such, you'll probably sign up for at least a month's worth of classes. Most teachers don't allow anything less and naturally they'll prefer more, but a month is a safe bet for most classes. If the class is everything you hope for, you'll re-up every thirty days by paying in advance for the next month.

Occasionally, you will fall in love with your acting teacher. I don't mean this literally. What I'm referring to is having an extraordinary instructor who helps you to grow in many ways as an actor. That's nice, but sometimes when that happens actors might find themselves never leaving this environment. That's not a good thing. You risk getting too comfortable. That place, although wonderful to visit, might ultimately make it harder in the outside world.

Although it might be tough to walk away from a great teacher, when you feel like you've learned everything you can from that person, it's probably time to move on. If you feel you're doing the same stuff repeatedly, or if you feel you aren't taking chances like you used to—chances that actually made you a better actor—then maybe it's time. Your teacher will understand and probably knew this well before you did.

The other end of the spectrum is the teacher who rules her class like a tyrant. Thankfully, those individuals are few and far between, but there are a rare few who make it their life's goal to rule over their students through head games, harassment, and generally abusive treatment. If you find yourself in such a classroom, there is an easy solution. Stop payment on your check and get the hell out of there.

In almost all cases, when you are studying on-camera, it will be a single camera in the classroom. That will suffice for most situations as that's the way it is on a real set. Sometimes they're shooting more than one camera but that shouldn't affect your performance. However, on certain shows, almost always sitcoms and daytime serials, they tape (as opposed to film) with multiple cameras on-set. These shows are often done in real time (or as close as they can without stopping). They are cut live and your cues will be completely different than on a standard film set. If you have the opportunity to get some practice in a three- or four-camera situation, do so. At the very least, watch a few tapings of sitcoms (they're free and always looking for seat fillers) and, if you have any chance to attend dress rehearsals or camera blocking rehearsals, do so. It'll prepare you for the first time in that unique area of television.

Actors

You'll share LA with actors all the time—you can't escape them. Throw a stick down La Cienega Boulevard and you'll hit five actors. Throw one down Radford and you'll hit ten. Actors are everywhere. They're auditioning alongside you, with you, and sometimes against you. Away from work, you'll meet them serving dinner at restaurants, biking along the beach, managing your apartment building, and hanging out at Starbucks, where by the way I'm writing this section, sitting not very surprisingly next to an actress pitching herself to a screenwriter perched right next to her.

This abundance of actors can get overwhelming at times. Remember when you thought acting was a *unique* profession? It might have been just that in Miami, Philadelphia, or Denver, but not here where the Department of Motor Vehicles is fresh out of any kind of vanity plate that has ACT in the spelling. For survival sake, I propose you accept the awesome presence around you, even be bemused by it, because it's not going to change as long as they're making movies in Hollywood.

Given the tremendous number of performers, and the inevitable scarcity of work, you will be quite happy to know that we actors coexist quite well overall. You'll generally like and appreciate those who share your profession. You'll meet real pros, establish friendships with some, and work with many others who will help and occasionally inspire you. Sure everyone is seeking out the work, but most don't step on each other or lose their dignity in trying to get it.

However, there are a few who will make you wish they'd identify themselves as something other than actors. There are the shameless promoters who buy billboards to splash their faces. Others will try to intimidate you at auditions. There are also performers who carry large chips on their shoulders, and more than a few who insist the industry is one giant conspiracy designed to keep them out. There are the clingers who trail you around sets. There are those who insist on never-ending name dropping. There are also the overcompetitive types who are so totally into themselves that they forget they're more than the work they seek. There are a whole bunch of head cases, probably as there are in all professions, but just a little more prevalent in ours. One of your jobs will be making sure you can survive some of the very people who do what you do—act.

My advice is simple. Steer clear of individuals who are trying to load negative thoughts upon you. As much as possible, avoid those actors who are overly jaded, overly negative, overly suspicious, overly egotistical, overly agendized, overly nagging, overly in need of meeting *your* agent . . . okay, stay away from people who are just "over."

Half of acting success is your mental state. When you're feeling better, you get better results. Surround yourself with people who share that attitude and you'll get even better results. Know that there are times when it may be better to just get out of the way.

There are, of course, times you can't get out of the way, and inevitably there are going to be occasional personality clashes when working with creative people. Occasional conflict and disagreements are fine—often they help make for a better project. Disrespect and lunacy are something else altogether.

But you've got to be pragmatic. This is your career after all.

One job I certainly wasn't going to walk away from had me sitting in a transportation wagon with another actor who after a few minutes grabbed the walkie talkie from the driver and yelled, "Hey we're in the cast and we're getting pissed off sitting down here. When the hell are you bringing us to the set!" Holy crap, I thought, this guy thinks he's speaking for me. Well, he wasn't. No worry, they were already aware of his rotten attitude. You think this guy was some pampered star of the show? No, he was a dayplayer like myself.

Ageism

The last time I checked we were all getting older. That's part of life and certainly a factor professional actors must consider on their survival journey. The fact is ageism; frankly, all the *isms* are rampant in the film and television industry. In corporate America if they fire someone and it can be proven there was age discrimination, a lawsuit is in the making. Not possible in the acting field.

They might decide you're too old for the part, but they don't openly share that information and they never will. They just don't cast you. If you thought of coasting past this section because you don't consider yourself *old,* then think about this. Hollywood old is a different old than the real world old. As with professional athletes, there is an accelerated age stigma that can greatly affect your career. When most actors hit their thirties, they'll see less work than those in their mid-twenties. At forty-five, many pine for the work they got at thirty-five, which was already less than what they got the decade before.

At *Backstage West*, I've gotten letters from actors in their early twenties complaining how all of the teenagers are getting *their* auditions. Ageism is a factor for all actors, even those cute child actors who suddenly find themselves turning into teenagers. Nonstar actors in their 50s and 60s turn up so rarely on network television that you're almost startled when one appears. Hollywood does not often reward past excellence.

So I focus on ageism over the other isms because it is truly the one we all share and must deal with. How then do you survive growing older in Hollywood? Each year you age you have to work that much harder to not let them forget you. It can be done. It has to be done.

It seems every two years or so the Screen Actors Guild spends a good-size chunk of its members' money to do yet another study on sexism, racism, and ageism. The results are always the same. Women are hired much less than men. Caucasians are employed much more than minorities, and younger actors get many more work days than older ones.

I'm optimistic and hope that someday those numbers will become more balanced, but for all its progressive reputation things are very slow to change in Hollywood. Young isn't just a trend, it's a perceived need. Some have decided that the typical viewer, and therefore the person that entertainment should be designed for, is a fourteen-year-old boy with the attention span of a hummingbird. Of course, every time a good feature film with a mature cast is released, it does incredible business and the wizards try to figure out from where all the old people came. Answer, they've always been there.

Nevertheless, most of the product that comes across the big screen and the small screen is designed for a young audience. For every "Gosford Park" there are a dozen "American Pies." It stands to reason that if the product is made for younger viewers the casts are going to represent that. Hollywood is famous for repeating itself. When *Friends* premiered and was a huge hit, you knew the next season would have a slew of clone shows, and there were. Most of them tanked.

So the casting skews younger. However, you must also consider this. Probably eight out of ten professional actors fall in that twenty-something age range. More roles are cast, but there are that many more candidates to fill them. For older actors there will likely be fewer auditions, but they'll also be facing that much less competition for the work. Now don't for a moment think that this will be the break you've been waiting for. There will still be plenty of competition, throughout the years regardless of your age. At "Tombudsman," I also hear from plenty of successful businessmen and women who are throwing their old careers away for a shot at being actors or actresses in Hollywood. Dreams of acting success are not solely the domain of the young set.

You can obsess about ageism, or you can accept it as one of those things you can't fully change and work that much more diligently in pursuit of your share of the pie. Recognize that ageism exists and if you're ever in a position to change it try and do so.

Don't volunteer your age. If you're fifty-five and you look forty-five, then your resume should state "age range 40–50." By the way, they should never ask your actual age; if they do, it's illegal. Just try to avoid that discussion because it really doesn't matter once you're over eighteen. In acting, you're only as old as you look.

Another way to fight the ageism bug is to keep yourself as young and fresh as possible. There are plastic surgery procedures that some go for, but that's not what I'm referring to. I'm talking *mentally* young and fresh. As the years progress, many veteran actors tend to slow down on their marketing and that other thing that actors do in their earlier years—always thinking of ways to reinvent and reinvigorate themselves. You can't allow that to happen. Whether you're thirty, forty, fifty, or eighty years of age for that matter, there's always something new to do, a better approach, or a new take on the situation, always new classes, new pictures, or a new agent or manager. Get yourself in that mind-set once again. Make your new age an asset. Remember that they need cast members in all ages. If you're the best actor in your category, still marketing aggressively and taking care of yourself physically, you're likely going to be the actor who gets a good amount of those available roles.

Agents

Everybody who arrives in Hollywood says the same thing. "How do I get an agent?" Many should perhaps be saying, "How do I get in acting class," but they get their priorities all twisted around. Indeed so influential and sought after are agents that many a discombobulated newcomer seeks one out long before his skills will make him an attractive candidate to one. In short, you want an agent when having one will be beneficial for both you and the agency.

Can you survive in LA without an agent? Can you breathe without oxygen? Not for long. The good news is, in the short term anyway, you certainly can at least get started and maybe even land some professional work without an agent. Between smaller parts on television shows, theatre roles, lower-budget commercials, and independent film gigs, there are ample audition opportunities for a hustling actor who is without a talent representative. Those jobs will help lead you to your first agency. So don't fret when you hear that you'll perish in Los Angeles without an agent, because as an aggressive and focused actor you'll survive without one, at least for a while.

Ultimately, to get any type of consistency and upward direction in your career, you'll eventually need an agent. A great one would be nice, but you'll probably be very lucky to find a good one. Many actors stop worrying about landing a big one when they realize the huge number of Los Angeles performers also seeking representation. Then they madly rush for any agency that'll have them. You definitely want an agent, but you don't want to be desperate and sign with someone you feel could be detrimental to your career. Unfortunately, you usually find these things out after the fact. Be as smart as you can be and know that you can always find a way to move on if things aren't clicking.

Whatever the size of the agency, what matters most is honest representation from someone who is going to push you forward and open some doors. You'll need to find an agent who is actually going to do something for you beyond piling your headshots in a filing cabinet. When you find that agency, you'll be on your way to building a career. This all takes time. You can't expect to take the town by storm. If it happens, great, but don't be foolish enough to plan a career around it. Like any business you play it smart, stay aggressive, and don't waste your opportunities. An agent will be watching to make sure you don't.

You'll need an agent's advice, guidance, contacts, and ultimately their state-licensed ability to negotiate a contract once you've booked a job. California licenses all its talent agencies and grants them the right to handle all paperwork related to you working as an actor. This is the major difference between an agent and a manager.

There are two types of agents you'll primarily be looking for and working with as a Los Angeles actor. The *theatrical agent* represents performers for film and television roles, which is the toughest area in which to find auditions for an actor. It's not surprising then that getting a theatrical agent is a very difficult task, but it can be done.

A *commercial agent* is somewhat easier to land as this agent represents many more actors and is usually receptive to performers who aren't with an already strong resume. Keep the word "easier" in perspective. It's still difficult to find one who'll sign you.

Theatrical and commercial agents account for most of the jobs casting, but there are also agents who represent performers for theatre work, stunt jobs, dancing, voice-overs, and pretty much any other specialty in the entertainment world. If you hope to work in multiple areas, you will seek someone to assist you in each one.

Within the talent agency ranks are many levels and sublevels. There are the one-person operations that cater to newer or less-credited actors, boutique agencies that have perhaps a few to a half-dozen agents and a relatively small client list, and the mid-size entities that employ even more agents and subagents and have multiple departments as well as a wide array of working actors in their files. Of course, there are also the few well-publicized superstar agencies that are nearly as powerful as some of the studios, and they won't even be interested in helping you get work until you've already gotten plenty of it yourself.

Don't waste your time calling the last guys. Rest assured, when you have your name on a contract as a series' regular, they'll miraculously find you. But let's not put the cart before the horse.

If you're like most actors, as the years pass, you'll climb the ladder up through the different agency levels. The majority of performers start somewhere near the bottom, and only a few ever make it to one of the powerhouse agencies that package their clients—writers, directors, and actors—into many of the major films and television shows.

You needn't be with a so-called super agency to have a good career. In fact, most never get to those big three or four. There are countless examples of actors who have been signed with small or medium-size agencies for years and had respectable working careers. Some have gotten a big part and moved upward only to eventually return to their old agency after finding less attention paid to their career from the behemoth that promised them the stars.

Casting director Lisa Miller Katz, of CBS's "Everybody Loves Raymond," deals with agents big and small on a daily basis and observes,

> The truth of the matter is, it's not that the bigger agencies always do more and the smaller agencies don't. It's very rare to me that there is an actor out there who is one hundred percent happy with their representation. Whether it's a huge agency or a small one most actors feel they're not getting sent out enough. That's a given, but it's much more the slightly small boutiquey agencies where I feel the agents really know, love and respect their clients.

The bottom line is that a good agent is a good agent, whatever their address, but you cannot ignore that the bigger agencies wield most of the power in Hollywood. If during your career you have the opportunity to sign with one of these people, you will no doubt take it. The actors at the largest agencies aren't necessarily better, but they certainly get the major share of the auditions for the better roles.

For now, let's operate on the assumption that, like most average actors, you're not currently entertaining an offer from the William Morris Agency.

A new actor has his choice of a few dozen agencies that handle newcomers. These first-level agencies wield little power, are usually one- or two-person operations, and at best are a stepping stone in an actor's career. These agents know, are comfortable with it, and are never shocked when their busier clients leave them to move up the line. But getting an agent at even this level is tough. There are so many talented actors dying to be seen by anyone that even the smallest agency is inundated with strong potential clients. Where does that leave you if you have few or no credits? Unless you are extraordinarily beautiful or handsome, you'd probably do better trying to find student and low-budget independent films, theatre, and other accessible casting possibilities on your own rather than going full tilt with agency mailings. This can be a time when it's better to be nonunion because much of the smaller projects are not done under union contracts. Try to score some work opportunities to build your resume. This will make you a more attractive candidate to agencies.

Some actors sign with their first or second agency and are happy to stay with them for many years. If you're busy and working, and understand that most actors aren't so fortunate, you might remain right where you are. However, when things slow down, actors are known to start looking around for greener pastures.

Actors ask themselves the inevitable questions. Why are other people working? Why can't I even get an audition? What's the reason I'm not being submitted for certain shows that I'm perfect for? The answers often lead to a search for a new talent representative.

Newer actors to town usually get their first agency appointment through sheer hard work that usually comes in the form of a mass mailing. It's not glamorous work, but if you put enough envelopes in the mail you'll eventually get some response. There might be better ways to meet an agent—a personal recommendation from another actor or perhaps a representative from the office seeing you in a play can lead to a meeting—but when push comes to shove many performers rely on 8×10s, manila envelopes, and postage as their primary method of agent seeking.

When it lands on an agent's desk, your picture will be lucky to get a glance that lasts longer than a few seconds. If it isn't tossed immediately, then he may flip it over to look at your resume. If you survive that turnover (and many don't), it may be put into a file that includes lots of other pictures of actors who may or may not ever be called in for a meeting. Every office and each agent within it works a little different. One may have his assistant phone an actor immediately after he gets the shot. Another will collect all possible candidates and make a few calls on a weekly basis. It comes down to what time of year and what the agency's needs are at the current time. The same actor could do fantastic in June and terrible in September. It's not a science; if the first mailing doesn't work, do another one in the not-too-distant future.

The owner of the Bobby Ball Talent Agency, Patty Grana-Miller, reveals the usual methods of getting seen by agents. "There are a few basic ways. Mailed submissions are very common, however, they are less effective than live showcasing (theatre, improv, etc.) or a personal introduction to an agent whether it be from a casting director or a current client we represent."

After the headshots go out, actors inevitably wonder whether they should follow-up with a phone call. I'm not going to declare you shouldn't call sometime later to see if they have your picture, but here is the answer you're probably going to get: "I don't see your picture, but someone will call you from the office if we're interested."

Have I ever broken this rule and called to follow-up? Sure. Has it ever worked? Only once. The person who answered told me she didn't recognize my name and that I should send another to her directly. I did and got an appointment. That time it worked, but usually it doesn't.

The good news is that they actually will call if they're interested. The bad news is that they *aren't* usually interested, and it's nothing personal but even the smallest agency, even one with just a so-so reputation, will get dozens of headshots every day. They have a lot to choose from.

Your first encounter with an agent will likely be a humbling experience. Chances are you'll be meeting someone in a very small office. The person might appear overworked and probably won't be able to give you more than a few minutes of his time. If the agency has a receptionist you'll be brought in; otherwise, you'll meet the front desk person who is also the subagent, agent, owner, and plant waterer.

In other words, it'll probably be a one- or two-person show. If you're sensible, you'll thank your lucky stars you've gotten this far. Don't ever treat a small agency as anything less than appropriate for where you are in your career. If you do, you can bet that the actor with a good attitude who visits the agency after you will look all the much better.

If you've come to Los Angeles with some strong regional credits, or if you've already been working here and are seeking a new talent representative, your chances of being seen by a medium-size agency or one of the stronger boutiques increase. Always be pragmatic and try to identify the agencies that are most likely to bring in an actor of your level—talentwise, creditwise, and otherwise.

You can easily identify the possibilities by reading one of the books that discusses specific agencies—*The Agencies* is a popular book that is published monthly—and by listening to other actors in class who know the agency reputations and preferences very well.

Patty Grana-Miller has this to say on the issue of agency size and attractiveness:

> I think it's a chemistry. It could be that one-man office who works tremendously well for you and if you went to some huge agency you'd be lost, or vice-versa. You have to go in with an open mind and do your homework no matter what size they are. If you have credits you know the business well enough to know whether or no that person is going to be able to work well for you and have a handle on who you are.

Whatever agency calls you in for an interview, you're going to be sitting in a chair across from a man or a woman who might be able to kick your career up a notch. That's important, but you can't let it wrack your nerves or cause you to hyperventilate. This is just one of many people you'll meet throughout the years. Do the best you can and like everyone always says quite correctly—be yourself. That's who they want to see. You know your own personality, your strengths and selling points. If you like to talk, then chat it up, but don't force yourself to be cute, overly talkative, or anything that isn't natural to the real you, and above all, don't be desperate. You've already won. They chose your headshot from among the many that they have received. So enjoy the experience, whatever the end result.

Often the early part of the meeting will be about your background, where you came from, what you hope to do, who you know (which for newer actors will probably be no one, but that's okay), your credits, etc. Then they'll tell you what their agency is all about and, if things are going exceedingly well, how they see you fitting in there.

Unlike what you may have experienced in New York or other places, no one here will ask you to do a monologue. When I arrived in 1994, like most actors I had a handful of solo scenes I could pull out for all occasions but soon found that they just weren't requested by LA film and television agents. You may very well read, especially for a commercial agent, but it will be from a script or sides—all the better to approximate how you'll do when you're standing in front of a casting director or producer.

Theatrical agents are more likely to give you a nice interview and then look at your demo reel, although some will throw you a page or two from a television show or film script to read. If they saw you on stage prior to the meeting, you've already sealed the deal and may not be asked to do anything. Though agents in LA are focused on film and television, they certainly want you to have theatre credits because it shows you are a dedicated professional. Even so they need to see what your skills are when reading for television and film parts, and monologues don't apply.

Commercial agents will give you one to several pieces of copy, allow you some time in the outer office to rehearse, and then bring you in. Most do this before they interview you. If you read the stuff to their liking, they'll then give you the full interview similar to a theatrical agent. Keep in mind when any agent is meeting you they are not only evaluating your talent but also your marketability. Your picture, resume, and reel have obviously answered a lot of those questions, but they'll never get the full picture until they have you in front of them. If you give a great commercial read and don't get selected by the agency, it could be for a million reasons. More often than not it's simply because they already have someone or several clients already in your type.

If you are what they're looking for, you'll hear the magic words—"We'd like to work with you." Normally, a one-year contract will be offered to the union performer and very often a longer-term agreement is put before the nonunion performer. On occasion, an agent may want to work without a contract to test the waters with an actor. If you are offered a contract, I recommend that you take it home and study it before signing. However, in their exuberance, many actors grab the first pen they can find to make it official. No reputable agency will mind if you take the contract with you. You must make sure you are crystal clear on what areas you are signing for—theatrical or commercial, or *across the board*—in which case the agency would submit you for auditions in both of those areas combined. The contract will also spell out the specifics of the agency responsibilities and what you're responsible for.

Your agency will undoubtedly have you fill out size cards, client information sheets, check authorization forms, and all types of written material. Then comes the next step, which is you supplying your new agent with headshots and resumes. During your meeting, you will have shown your pictures to the agent and she would have probably picked out one to three. These are the ones you'll need to furnish them with as soon as possible. Do not keep your agency waiting for pictures at any time during your relationship. If they don't have headshots on file, you might miss the one audition that can make a real difference.

Over time you'll find out how your agency works. Each one is different. You'll learn how much marketing they expect you to continue to do on your own behalf, what their preferences are for staying in touch and stopping by, and which agents and personnel are your day-to-day contacts at the office.

If you find a strong agency that stays motivated about you and your career, you will have many positive months and years ahead of you. The right agent can indeed make all the difference between working and not working. You'll have to deliver the goods when they get you in the door, but with their assistance it becomes a door easier opened. Your agent will pitch you to casting directors of projects that you're right for and appointments will eventually come. How many auditions you get and what happens from them will ultimately define the longevity of your relationship with the agency. In the best-case scenario, you'll have all the results you hope for and will build a lasting partnership. However, if things don't turn out as well as you hoped, there are always other agencies to consider. Most actors have been with more than a few.

If you're like most performers, you'll be associated with potentially many agencies through the years. You'll find honest, hardworking individuals who work tirelessly and ethically on your behalf. If, however, you find yourself at an agency that doesn't seem to fit that bill, you owe it to yourself to ask questions. If you don't get the right answers, you cannot ignore the writing on the wall. Although it's never easy to get an agent, you'd be far worse off with one that isn't doing their job—or worse, isn't on the up and up—than with none at all. Choose wisely and whenever possible, deal with the agencies that until recently, anyway, were franchised.

In April 2002, the long-standing agreement between the two major talent agency organizations—the Association of Talent Agents (ATA) and the National Association of Talent Representatives (NATR)—and the Screen Actors Guild (SAG) officially ended. Before then a SAG member was only able to work with one of these franchised agencies. Because SAG membership voted against recent agreement changes as we stand today, the atmosphere is one of much confusion. SAG members are still allowed to work with their formerly franchised agencies, but SAG has told them it is permissible to do so as long as agencies don't offer new contracts that are different than the standard agreements. There is much discussion about increased commissions and whether SAG members will at some point be forced to choose between their union and their agencies. In July 2002, the industry was pretty much in a "wait and see who'll make the next move" mode. This issue appears to be heading for a fall showdown.

Attitude

I'm really happy that attitude begins with the letter "A," because it'll cause you to read this section before getting into the rest of the book. You need all the actor tools that we're so familiar with—headshots and resumes, demo reels, training, and talent—to get anywhere in Hollywood.

Just as you'll require those things, so will you need to keep a positive attitude from day to day. This is a challenging business in which to do that, but the failure to do so has caused the downfall of some very good performers. Don't let it happen to you. I'll talk about some of the most common undesirable attitudes later in the book; however, for now I want to discuss the good attitude, because it's the one that will help your career, not hinder it.

So much of your success is going to be dictated by what goes on in your head. You have a choice each day, either get up and attack the acting business with passion, relish, and positivity, despite the obvious toughness of the field, or just become one of those people that progressively gets angrier and watches it erode their work *and* their art.

That's the key. What we do is both work and art combined. As a professional actor in Los Angeles, you cannot hide one from the other. If you have a bad attitude about the business, it will inevitably show up in your demeanor at auditions and meetings. It won't show up in work, because you won't get that far. A good attitude will open doors and expand your horizons professionally. If you watch employed professionals—not just stars but everyday working actors—their attitude is usually positive about the art and the commerce. That's the professional acting business. This doesn't mean you march in blindly, smiling and accepting everything you see. You're a professional actor, and you must approach your field pragmatically, intelligently, and sometimes questioning when things aren't being handled properly. You can do this with a good attitude.

Auditions

I'll cover the different types of auditions (television, film, commercials) crucial to an actor in LA in their own A–Z areas. Yet, there needs to be some discussion of auditioning in general because most of your time as a performer consists of two things—waiting for auditions and actual auditioning.

Unless you're a major name actor, and sometimes even then, you will have to audition for nearly every role you want to play. You must learn to be a consistently good, if not great, auditioner to have an ongoing career in Hollywood. Although casting directors often have great memories, it usually comes down to "what have you done for me lately." You may have worked for someone a few times in the past, but they still need you to be solid in the audition today before they'll bring you in to the people that might hire you tomorrow.

You might be a wonderful actor who just isn't a good auditioner, but if you can't get past the casting director, the director, and the producers and writers during the audition process you may never make it to an actual set. You've got to come to terms with auditions and make them work for you. Training, experience, and time will make you a better auditioner but even that isn't always enough.

Brian Myers, one of the casting directors on arguably the most successful sitcom ever—"Seinfeld"—and who currently casts NBC's "Just Shoot Me" and "Watching Ellie," explains:

> Nobody does it exactly the same way, but a lot of people come in and interpret the material similarly. You see a lot of people doing a variation of the same thing and then someone will do something different, and that actor stands out. What often works, is a strong choice but an appropriate choice.

To make that happen you have to get in there and do it a few times. When you aren't glued to the page, intimidated by the people in front of you, or afraid to take that strong but appropriate choice, you take one huge step forward in your career. The good news is you'll grow with each audition, and you may even learn to enjoy the process.

You still have to go on a lot of auditions to get a little work. Supply and demand again! The odds are always unfavorable, but a realistic actor accepts that and works with it. How you deal with the process is a reflection of your experience. At first, you'll carry around an audition that didn't go well for a week or two, replaying over and over what you should have done differently. You might have been perfectly fine, but you'll still find one thing—maybe a word—that you didn't think you nailed and you'll obsess on it. Then magically one day you won't.

You'll always have a little replay time, but a professional learns to let auditions fly away in a reasonable time frame. You have to, because another fact of the television and film world is that many times when you don't get the part, or sometimes when you do, it may have little to do with your actual acting. Your nose, your height, your accent, or your resemblance to the writer's annoying brother can all lead to you not being cast, or being cast for that matter. All you can do as an auditioning actor is to be as prepared as possible and let them see what you would do with the part should they be smart enough to hire you. Then go have a Starbucks.

Avoiding Scams

There's no doubt about it, when things are going well for an actor in Los Angeles, it can be the greatest place on earth. The sun is perpetually shining, you find yourself hired on a show working with wonderful and supportive people, and there's always the potential for a career-making role, right around the next soundstage. Los Angeles can embrace you and nurture you, but it can also show you its uglier side from time to time.

There are so many scams perpetrated on actors in this city that you'd sometimes think the whole place is one giant rip-off waiting to happen. I cannot think of one other profession and city in which charlatans, crooks, and manipulators exist in such high numbers.

There are some well-placed boosters and political types in this metropolis who refuse to even acknowledge show business problems exist. Problems do exist, and actors have to find ways to keep them at arm's length by their own wits.

You can accomplish scam avoidance if you're smart, day in and day out. Never let your common sense be clouded by offers that are too good to be true. You must remember that you are in a real business, not a fairy tale. Otherwise, sensible people get sucked in when someone seemingly in a position of power delivers an attractive pitch. Don't swing! Showbiz con artists take advantage of newcomers and some not-so newcomers by promising the keys to the kingdom if you pay them, please them, or do anything for them that would be considered unacceptable or illegal in the real world. People that are alert to possible rip-offs have successful careers, and the crooks steer clear of them in favor of more gullible and vulnerable prey.

LA is a city that welcomes the dreamer, and many who do get conned, ripped off, or worse just keep their mouths shut for fear that speaking out will somehow harm their career. This is nonsense, but that attitude has persisted for years and has only encouraged crooks to focus on those who are looking for some way, any way, to make it as actors.

A popular scam, unpopular for the victims, involves companies that pitch themselves as some type of talent representative. Great, the actor thinks, an agency that wants me! Once the actor goes in for the interview, he finds he is required to pay an upfront or sometimes monthly fee for this representation. Legitimate talent agents and managers only take a commission for booked work. They don't require any advance fees, and they won't insist you take their classes, use their in-house photographer, or go away with them for a long weekend in Las Vegas. This is common knowledge, yet every day several people pay someone posing as a talent representative large amounts for some promise of future employment. Don't do it.

That's probably the most common everyday scam, but if there is another way to cheat an actor someone is out there doing it. Some scammers are fly-by-nighters and others have been doing it so long they have well-established offices around town. Snakes come in all colors and sizes, so don't be swayed by a pretty office, a wall full of star headshots, or a tantalizing pitch.

Thankfully, victims have begun to get more aggressive in going after crooks, and aided by information sharing over the Internet, actors are smarter and more well-informed than ever before. A growing campaign by the city attorney's office to help shut down entertainment scams is slowly but surely making the landscape look brighter for actors.

Mark Lambert is the Los Angeles Deputy City Attorney and has been involved in many prosecutions of those who would rip off actors. He speaks about some of the scams going on and what performers must do to help themselves:

> Most scams happen to newcomers. Someone will induce an actor or actress to pay money up front for either photos, or classes in order to be your manager or agent. It's against the law. If that happens, the best thing for you to do is make a complaint to the Los Angeles County Department of Consumer Affairs. If it's a sex crime or something like that, you should first call directly to the police. Our office is a prosecuting office, not an investigative one. Consumer Affairs will investigate and if they find merit they'll bring it to our office for possible criminal filing. The most important thing actors need to do is make the complaint. Too many times they get ripped off and just decide it's a learning experience or nobody will help them. However, when the complaints add up, that's when things happen. By not complaining you're letting them keep your money and basically cheat other people the same way. You should document things, write things down when it's fresh in your mind. Actors shouldn't fear reprisals from these guys who are just scammers. They have no influence.

Influence is something an aggressive scammer will always try to make you think he has in spades. They know that most inexperienced people won't call their bluff or do any research.

Do the proper research and you may never experience any of the following events. The following instances are but a few of the hundreds we've heard about at *Backstage West*:

> From the "Tombudsman" files, there was one particularly stupid crook who tried to convince us that she was a respected producer for a major studio in Hollywood. She certainly tried to gain influence by dropping all the right names to the many actors who came in her office and ended up paying her for representation. It turns out, and this probably won't shock you, she was a classic crook playing the long con. When she finally returned our repeated calls at the paper, this wired A-type seemed to believe her own lies. She insisted we call one of the production heads at the studio to confirm she was who she said she was. We gladly obliged. With her on the other line, I called the studio person who promptly told us this imposter had nothing to do with the studio or the film she claimed to be producing. After the studio guy hung up, she nonchalantly told us that he was just mistaken. She was the producer is all she kept saying. The next call went to the star's agent. The agent knew all too well about this pest and said that there was no professional relationship between his client and this wacky-sack. Once the agent hung up, she started railing that the agent didn't

know what she was talking about either. This pathological liar had an answer for everything and that had helped her rip off countless young actors who wanted a part in some fictitious film she was supposedly heading up. However, no one was checking up on her as we were, and the victims were piling up by the day.

How do you think she has gotten away with this for years and is probably still out there conning people in new ways every day? One, she rented a nice suite on a good street in Beverly Hills. Two, she had the gift of rapid-fire BS, common among con artists. Third, she knew her victims were desperate for success and told them what they wanted to hear. Ultimately, she continued to get away with her exploits, as do many others today, because actors didn't call her on it.

If someone ran up to you and stole your purse, you'd call the cops. When someone claiming to be legit rips you off, why would you even consider not taking action?

Just to show you how crazy and stupid crooks are, let me tell you about the last thing I heard on this one. Several months later an actress called me to say she'd been in to interview with a movie producer—the same crook—who wanted her to pay her some money. And the producer was actually handing out copies of the article we'd written about her rip off, but she claimed we'd done a nice story about her. We'd written about her, but it wasn't nice.

If you're an actor for long enough, eventually someone will try to scam you. Nine out of ten times, it will be to get your money and perhaps the other time will be someone trying to get you in bed. There are still cases of innocent, and sometimes not so innocent, actors ending up on their back in promise of a role. "Hey, it worked for Marilyn" (or fill in another more recent celebrity name) the crook will claim, and too many confused, desperate young actors take the bait.

- There's the guy with a video camera and a room at his brother's house who is casting his feature film. He doesn't want you to get nude. Yet, he auditions you and tells you he wants you for your part. Oh, and one more thing, about the fee...the one you'll be paying to help produce the project.

- There's the supposed manager in Santa Monica, who has just moved to Beverly Hills, and then back to Santa Monica again (scammers tend to move around a lot for obvious reasons). His MO was to bring in actors and charge them for pictures, put them on his worldwide web site, and print their pictures at a discount. He also claims to represent some of the biggest names in television. The problem is he doesn't represent anyone but his own interests. In the end, the pictures never come, the representation doesn't represent, and your check for pictures, reprints, web site representation, and overall career *management* has cleared the bank.

- There's the guy who posted casting notices all over town seeking actresses for his independent film. The women show up and, if you make the callback, he asks you to disrobe so he can wrap your nude body in cellophane! This is not a joke. The stock in cellophane goes up in Los Angeles, but the guy disappears before the cops raise an eyebrow.

- There's a producer who regularly browbeats actors and practically jumps the bones of any nubile hopeful who has the misfortune of walking into his office. His bungalow is actually on a major studio lot. When the cops finally get a load of this jokester's ploys (he's only been doing it for ten years), they clandestinely remove him from their jurisdiction by means of secretive measures. The producer never realizes why his lease wasn't renewed. Nevertheless, without the legitimate guise of being on a real lot, he sets up shop a few miles away and goes right back to his nasty business. He's a great producer all right; even if he hasn't produced anything that you'd ever show your parents.

- There's the company that rips off starstruck parents and their excited children, charging them thousands of dollars on useless classes and materials that have little or no relation to the real business. Most of these victims are so shaken, embarrassed, and broke by the time they've been through the mill that they usually disappear without uttering a word to law enforcement.

Some newer actors are afraid to make waves; however, I urge you to make waves. Any threatened risk to your career is so outweighed by your duty to protect yourself and your dignity that you must not take it. Stand up for yourself as a professional actor.

Should something happen to you, Deputy City Attorney Lambert reminds you:

> The City Attorney's office has been aggressive in prosecuting these cases over the last several years and we will continue to be. We promise that we'll continue to look out for actors getting scammed as long as the actors let us know what's happening.

That's a promise that actors, who also happen to be registered voters, will be keenly watching. The number for the Los Angeles County Department of Consumer Affairs is (800) 593-8222. It's a toll-free call and a service paid for by taxpayers dollars.

I also suggest two other methods of scanning for scammers. The Better Business Bureau has a web site on which you can easily check up on any company you'd like to investigate. Go to www.search.bbb.org/results.html and simply put in the name of the company. If your hit brings back numerous complaints against a person or business, you should avoid them like the plague. Price for this service? Free again.

Also, scan a few of the actor chat rooms available around Los Angeles for information sharing. Now, you've got to take some of the stuff you read online with a grain of salt, but you'll see certain names over and over again that will help you avoid the well known rip-off artists in our industry.

Let me leave this section with a positive note. I'm really happy to report that crooks represent only a small fraction of the people you'll encounter during your time in Los Angeles. They are so outnumbered by the ethical people in our industry that you needn't ever let them distress you to the degree that you lose sight of the fact that there is much more good than bad in our field. You may be really lucky and never meet any of them. That is, if you're smart, tough when you need to be, and learn one magic word, "no," you will fair well.

B

Background Work

Also known as extra work, atmosphere work, or hell on earth depending on the particular set, background employment is everything you've heard of and more. It's also a great place to begin one's on-camera career. Where else can you gain valuable experience on a real set, be paid for your time, meet and mingle with actors and technicians, and sometimes get a bump into the glorified world of a speaking part?

It's also a cushion where veteran actors can pick up a few days work here and there to pay the bills and keep health benefits intact during those down cycles when the principal work just isn't coming. You won't hear experienced actors talking much about their extra jobs, but they do them.

Background performers generally fall into two categories. There are the professional extras who make their living through this type of work. Many of them have no desire to move up the ladder to speaking roles and are content in the knowledge that they get more on-set employment than many actors. They've found a way to make a nice living in a very tough business.

Some within this group work wherever and whenever they can get a gig—a drama here, a sitcom there, and occasionally they'll land a commercial extra job that pays a lot more than doing the same thing on a television show or film. The elite of background players might latch onto a regular background job on a series that lasts for years. You've seen shows where the same group of people are floating around the law office or coffee shop week after week, year after year—those are the happiest extras you'll ever find. Some even get bumped up to a speaking role from time to time.

The second category of backgrounders are those actors who have perhaps larger career aspirations. They are the performers who usually play or hope to play speaking roles, but sometimes find they need to fill in during the slow periods by doing some extra work. Many in this group refuse to consider themselves extras, although they'll gladly take the paycheck. They never list the work on their resumes for fear someone who casts the show's principal parts will see it and never bring them in to read for a speaking part.

This is a city where some people who haven't worked in years loudly proclaim, "Don't do extra work if you're serious about your career." That's baloney. Go check out a set and see who is doing the background work. You'll recognize plenty of familiar faces from the ranks of principal actors. But it's not just you saying you're going to do it that translates into getting a job.

Like in all categories of acting, there is only so much work to go around, especially if you're a union actor. Many of these performers were members of the Screen Extras Guild (SEG) when it existed. Now that SEG is long gone, its extras are under the jurisdiction of SAG. Holding a membership card in SAG, although paying you a higher wage than a nonunion performer, often means less work opportunity overall. Here's why.

Each day in Hollywood, the lion's share of people who are working as extras are nonunion performers. SAG and the American Federation of Television and Radio Artists (AFTRA) have contractually allowed producers to hire a large number of nonunion players after they meet their union quota on sets. The numbers might vary depending on the budget of a project, but generally a film producer who is a SAG signatory must hire forty-five union extras before he can open the gates to the nonunion performers. If you see a crowd scene, you can be assured the mass is primarily made up of nonunioners. For television shows, it's fifteen union hired before nonunion; for commercials, they must hire thirty-five union extras first. This all means that producers save big money because nonunion extras get at best about one half the pay and less perks.

It's been suggested that a lot more union actors might consider extra work if there was work available to them. Nonunion actors can get very busy doing background while making a decent wage. Eventually they may collect three union vouchers, which will gain them entry into SAG.

The vouchers, which guarantee the nonunion actor a union wage, are disbursed when one of the required union members doesn't show for work. An assistant director will then give that voucher to any nonunion actor of his choosing. This creates plenty of jockeying as the nonunion people are always trying to stay in the good graces of an assistant director who might reward them with a voucher. When three vouchers are collected, the actor can join SAG. It also might mean actually working less because he's part of SAG now and potentially losing work to a nonunion actor like his former self.

Depending on your goals—short and long term—you might map out a sensible plan for doing extra work. If you are looking at principal roles as your big picture career plan, then you do not want anyone to think you are focused on background work. Most people wouldn't anyway. Casting directors know that actors survive by doing some occasional extra work. Agents know that their newer, and sometimes older, clients occasionally dip their toes in the background waters. No one really cares. However, they'll care very much if they're trying to get you a recurring or regular role on a series while you're doing extra work on the show, but those cases are few and far between.

The fact is, you can do extra work to survive, and no one will be the wiser. It's not a subject that ever comes up at an audition. Savvy actors take the work for what it is—a chance to get some tuning and a paycheck. If, however, you are serious about playing principals, you would never choose a day's work as a background performer over attending an audition for a principal role. You must prioritize.

A performer who is content being a full-time background actor might list a ton of projects on their resume, but a principal player doing background work isn't going to include these credits on their resume. So, although industry people won't care if you squeeze in some amount of this work, don't highlight it on your resume or in mailings to casting directors.

If you are here for bigger things, you should probably do only as much background work as you need to survive. If you continue to do it beyond getting early experience or to pay those immediate bills, you could very well have it become your main career focus without even realizing it.

Another reason some people tell you to steer clear of extra work has nothing to do with its classification. It's sometimes just a tough environment to handle. It has gained and maintains its reputation as a thankless and sometimes depressing place in which to work. You could be faced with an assistant director who screams, having to work twelve- to fifteen-hour days, standing in the rain, getting baked in the hot sun, or you might find yourself stuck in a freezing cold holding area with no signs of life.

The caste system makes no sense to the newly arrived professional actor who happens to be doing a day's work as a silent performer so that he can maybe qualify for his health benefits. Yesterday he was playing Hamlet to an adoring audience, and today he's getting an earful from a production assistant fresh out of film school for taking a can of soda from the food table of a $90-million-budget film. Meanwhile, the actor standing next to him who is a one-line principal has been given a trailer and can eat anything he wants to from the same table.

If you do enough background work, you will find the stereotypically horrible set; yet, you could do a lot of this work and never have anything major occur. On most sets, extras are left alone, treated well, and earn a reasonable paycheck for walking past the camera a few times.

On some sets, it only takes one way-out background performer to cause grief for the whole lot. There are a few people who by their sheer bizarre behavior give all extras a bad reputation. Avoid these people and you'll be fine. Locate the professionals and hang around them. Let the assistant director know every time you leave the holding area to use the restroom and you'll be the hero. In the meantime, you'll find yourself working with actors you've seen on films and in television for years, while learning a lot about the hierarchy and mysteries of a working Hollywood set. If you're a seasoned pro who knows all that stuff already, you'll be glad for the overtime and placement just far enough away from the camera that no one will recognize you. If the director decides he wants an extra to yell "Pizza" and he picks you, you'll be upgraded to principal status. You'll praise the day they invented extra work. If someone barks at you just because you wouldn't sit in a smoke-filled room for sixteen hours in three inches of water, you'll swear extra work is the worst gig on the planet. Hang in there; the next one could be the best.

If you want to get into the background hiring loop, there are three things you should do after unpacking your bags in Los Angeles. Register with several of the companies that specialize in background performers. Many charge for their service ($15–$30 is common), which they say is for registration and photo fees to put you in their databases for future work. If the charge is much more than that, avoid it and move on to another company. Some actors might wonder why they have to pay any fee, but the practice is so entrenched now that it has become an accepted norm. If the thought of paying a fee rubs you the wrong way, don't do it. Instead, focus on one of the companies that does not charge a fee. There are plenty of them, too. A few of the companies actually tack on a percentage charge based on what you make. This royal treatment is reserved for the nonunion performer, because they would never get away with such highway robbery with union performers.

Most extra registration companies have at least one day a week when they register new people. Once you're in the files, one of two things will happen. You'll either get a call to show up for a day's work on a set, or you'll never hear from them again. That's why you register with more than one.

The second thing you do is send your picture and resume to all the soap opera extra casting offices since they do their background casting in house. There are a handful of daytime dramas shot in LA and you might score some work from them during your background years. There will never be a charge for this. Find the names of the appropriate background casters and mail your headshot directly to them.

The third thing you do is purchase a copy of a book titled *Extra Work for Brain Surgeons.* This spirited and honest appraisal of extra work will tell you everything you'll want to know about doing this kind of work in Los Angeles. I don't normally plug books, but this one is good.

One thing you should not do is respond to advertisements that are posted on telephone poles that say, "Seeking Extras for Upcoming Work." These are rip-offs. You might do best by tearing one off the pole and depositing it in the nearest garbage can, thereby saving some young newcomer a lot of grief.

Billing and Credits

Billing and credits are two closely related topics that have a lot of relevance to your career as an actor working in film and television. Where one starts and the other ends is something of a head-scratcher. Let me try to clear this up.

A *credit* is what goes on your resume. Your credits affect your quote (your pay rate), which in turn affects the size of your role and leads to better billing. This then translates to better credits on your resume. To add to the confusion, you should understand that a credit is sometimes also a billing, as in the case of guest star and costar, but it isn't in other instances like recurring or supporting.

A *billing* is how your name appears on a television screen or film print, yet, this is often referred to as the credit roll. Billing is negotiated with the producer, just like your salary and amount of days you'll be working.

Does this make sense? I didn't think so. Thus, let's discuss *credits* first. Credits, the right credits, count. You may have played Shakespeare stupendously in Central Park's Dellacorte; your Petruchio may have been perfect. However, on the resume of a working Los Angeles actor, a decent guest star role on a hot drama will usually carry a lot more practical weight for your day to day career.

Of course, some people who hire you are going to know and respect your theatre work. Others aren't even going to give those credits a passing glance on your resume, unless of course you starred with Nicole Kidman in "The Blue Room." They'll take notice of that.

Whatever their individual expertise and resume preferences, everyone in Hollywood zeros in on the credits under the headings of "Film" and "Television."

On top of that, they like to hire actors who are demonstrating current success, in other words, already working. You've heard the old expression, "It seems like the same people are working over and over again." That's true in many cases. If you have recent credits in film and television, you stand an excellent chance of getting even more auditions and, therefore, more credits.

Role size is important and, for the long-term career in Hollywood, bigger is definitely better. To progress upward, you must always be looking for more substantial roles. Larger roles afford the actor artistic growth and monetary enhancement. That doesn't mean you won't do one- or two-liners, even after you've played bigger parts, but the career objective for most actors is to move up the ladder when the opportunity presents itself.

From smallest to largest, this is how principal television roles break down creditwise. To help clarify the aforementioned credit/billing marriage, I'll designate each category as to whether it is generally considered a credit, C, or both a credit and a billing, B.

- *Featured* (C)—I'm hesitant to even include this credit, but it exists so here it is. I'm tentative because everyone has a slightly different view of what featured actually means. One person equates it with nonspeaking principal work, another believes it means one or two lines, and yet another views it as extra work with some special business. Whatever the case, the role is certainly very small. Once in a blue moon, you'll see "featuring" as a billing, but it's very rare.

- *Under-five* (C)—This is a category of hiring that is never heard of under SAG's contracts but is regularly used for AFTRA work, particularly in variety shows and daytime serials. It's pretty much how it sounds—if you are hired for this category, you will be speaking five lines or less. They also employ some nonspeaking actors but pay them as under-fives.

- *Costar* (B)—A costar is most often an actor hired by the day and occasionally for repeated days. In fact, much of the time you'll hear the category referred to as a dayplayer, though the credit at the end of the show falls under costar. The role sizes are varied anywhere from a few words like "Here's your pizza" to several pages of a long scene at which point the actor starts to wonder why she wasn't offered a guest starring part.

- *Also Starring* (B)—This is a billing you'll predominantly find on sitcoms. It represents a role that is of costar size, or it could be slightly larger than costar but is not a guest role. Again, this is no exact science because the term means one thing to one producer and something else to another.

- *Guest Star* (B)—A guest star role is almost always a meatier part that recurs throughout an episode—anywhere from three to several scenes would be a fair assumption. Look at an episode of "The Practice," for instance, and you can almost be guaranteed that the actor playing the main defendant of the week, who appears with the attorneys before, during, and after the trial, is a guest star. The actor playing the bailiff is undoubtedly a costar. Guest star roles pay more and get the actor better billing, which is very beneficial for future negotiations. It also can put the first-time guest star into a new category in the mind of the casting director.

- *Principal* (C)—This is a resume credit that I've only seen used by players on soaps and variety shows who are given more than five lines to speak.

- *Recurring* (C)—This is a credit you would be very fortunate to land. It means you are going to return for at least two and possibly several episodes in the same role. It could be as either a guest star or costar, but it's a return visit to a set and character. It's a nice step up the ladder for an actor. All the benefits go up as one would expect. There have been many cases when recurring guest stars have ended up moving into starring roles. A recurring guest role might be the sister of the lead who drops in every four or five weeks for some witty banter or it could be the costar cop who shows up every once in awhile at the squad house to drop off a perp to one of the series' handsome regulars.

- *Series Regular* (C)—The crème de la crème of television crediting. These are the starring cast members who have a season or hopefully many seasons of steady employment. Once you've starred on a show, you have reached a whole new level professionally and can start taking some real control of your career. If it's a hit, that is. However, if the show gets cancelled after three episodes (and that happens often), you're probably back on the pavement looking for that next pilot.

For the actors who make up the meat and potatoes of casts, newer credits go right on the resume, replacing the old ones. There are a hundred books that explain resume formatting for the Los Angeles actor, so I won't get into that here. Just know that your top credits—the largest parts from your most recent projects—should be somewhere near the top.

Now let's talk about the second part of this equation—the *billing* you'll be getting for your work.

Billings are used for a few purposes. First, they announce, on-screen, the stature or size of the role you are playing. They also help to determine your pay range for that project and how casters might ultimately see you for future work possibilities.

The theory is, the bigger the part, the earlier in the credit role, and the better the billing. For instance, a "top-of-show" guest star billing is something many middle-income earners strive for. Some shows, particularly one-hour dramas, offer top-of-show billing, and agents are always seeking these spots for their clients.

Top of show, especially when you have a separate billing card (your name alone on the screen for a couple of seconds), is considered better billing than a shared card (two or more names at the same time). Both of these placements are preferable to the guest star credit at the end of the show for two reasons. First, many people don't stick around for the final credits; second, networks are increasingly fond of squeezing the credits to the side of the screen to do promos for other programs.

Costar billing almost always happens quickly at the end of the show, so don't blink if you want to catch your name. Then again, if they squeeze it and speed up the roll, your name will look like hieroglyphics anyway. Don't worry too much about it. You did the gig and you got the credit.

Feature film billing and credits are much less complicated than those on television. In features, your on-screen billing will usually appear in the credits roll at the end. When your name is at the top of the film, you are doing very well and have an excellent agent. At the end, you'll either find your name in the classic "cast in order of appearance" manner or by role importance as determined by the director and producer.

As far as your resume is concerned, you'll almost always use the widely accepted "supporting" credit for any role size but the lead, in which case "starring" could go on your resume. As a working class actor, most of your roles will be anywhere from a line or two to several scenes, and supporting covers the bases quite well. Once you step it up further, the public and your agent will no doubt let you know when using "starring" is appropriate. Of course, you won't need a resume at that point either. I know nothing about this personally, but I hope to someday.

Breakdowns

As a professional actor, it won't be long before you'll become aware of the "Breakdowns." Breakdowns are the daily job listings released by casting directors, via the Internet, telling agents and managers what they are seeking castwise for films, television shows, commercials, theatre, and industrials.

They are also illegal for actors to receive or use as they are the copywritten property of a Los Angeles-based company called Breakdown Services, which aggressively protects its product. Yet many actors—neophyte through veteran—still buy the Breakdowns through one of the underground operations that sells them from coast to coast. Hungry actors are willing to take the chance that they won't get caught and that the rewards for taking that risk highly outweigh the negatives of possibly getting caught.

How do you survive this issue? Knowing the truth is a good place to start. Let's look at both sides of the issue.

Breakdown Services charges a fee to talent representatives to receive the listings each morning. It wasn't long ago (before the world wide web came into existence) that Breakdowns were faxed or delivered right to the door of the talent representatives. The reps go through the Breakdowns, which are essentially a Cliff Notes version of a script along with physical descriptions of the roles available, and decide which of their actors will be good candidates for specific parts. The reps then submit pictures and resumes of those actors to the appropriate casting director.

The whole system came into being in 1971 when an entrepreneur by the name of Gary Marsh discovered he could make life easier for the studios while ensuring a nice profit for his fledgling company. Prior to 1971, the casting directors and the studios for whom they worked had the arduous task of telephoning all over town to describe what they were looking for in terms of actors. Although he met some initial reluctance from the studios, Marsh's product ultimately made their life a lot easier. Thus, Breakdowns filled a huge need and after a few years took off into the dominant presence it is today.

Although many audition calls still come from connections between agents and casting directors that never even end up on a Breakdown, the fact is that thousands of projects, including many of the top shows, use Breakdowns on a daily basis to find the right actor for the role. There are approximately 600 agents and managers who pay to subscribe to these daily Breakdown lifelines to the casting world.

There are also significant numbers of actors who pay someone, other than Breakdown Services, to view what's being cast. As one actor told me, anonymously, for fear of being caught, "I'm going to do what I have to do. My agent doesn't get me enough work, and whenever I see the Breaks and send my own pictures I get more auditions. It's simple as that. I'll take my chances."

Those chances are not minimal, but let the owner of the company explain it in his words. According to Marsh, an amiable man who is despised by some actors who know nothing about him other than his name:

> The way the system works is, take an episodic television show. They've got maybe four days to cast it. The casting directors, even with the submissions they receive from the legitimate representatives of talent, are overwhelmed and don't open all of the submissions. If you add

actor submissions on top of that it's a case for anarchy when too many
people apply the "I'm right for the role" logic.

Marsh's theory about submissions numbers is all too correct. In
every casting director's office there are waist high stacks of freshly
arrived manila envelopes all holding headshots and resumes. Those
stacks make you realize you're lucky to get any audition in this com-
petitive town.

Still, actors are always looking for ways to get seen. As far as many
are concerned, any submission by any route, including the Breakdowns,
is better than sitting back and waiting. Some do it by purchasing the
Breakdowns illegally from a web of illegal sellers around Los Angeles.
How do these people find you? Well, your pager might go off one day
and a stranger is offering to sell you some goods. Chances are he's
not selling health insurance. Other times, it's an actor in class who
tells you he has source. There are many avenues. Some actors have
formed phony management companies (a few of which have evolved
into real management) to try and get the Breakdowns under the guise
of legitimacy. In general, to secure the product legally, an agency must
be either state licensed or a management company needs three letters
of recommendation from the owners of talent agencies.

Marsh is always on the lookout for individuals who are trying to
get the product illegally, but he's clear on who he sees as the crook and
who is the victim:

> My beef is not with the actor that is trying to get ahead. My beef is
> with the individual who preys on the actor and extracts cash from
> them in order to get access to the information. I know there are quite
> a few actors that have somehow managed to get the Breakdowns but
> I think it's buyer beware. These are basically stolen goods. It is illegal.
> There was one organization that violated my copyright and was fined
> a quarter of a million dollars and there are a couple of individuals
> that actually did jail time. Again my beef is not with the actor but
> with the person soliciting the actors. We have to protect our business;
> otherwise it gets out of hand. There is a perception in this town that I
> made some kind of nefarious decision to withhold information from
> actors. Obviously, if I could sell to actors I could make a lot more
> money than I do now.

Marsh also sets the record straight about going after individual actors. "I cannot condone their behavior because it ultimately is buying
stolen goods, but in the thirty years I've been in business I've never
prosecuted a receiver of Breakdowns."

Sellers certainly aren't going to get the same treatment. Marsh also
wants actors to know that his web site, www.breakdownservices.com/
access.html, does offer some Breakdowns (free of charge) that casting
directors have specifically requested actors have access to.

Burn Out

Burn out happens to all too many people in this difficult business. It's never easy to maintain your balance in a field that tests your mettle on a daily basis, but the surviving actor finds a way to make the instability and the uncertainty bearable. Most manage to do it.

For many though, it sometimes is just too overwhelming. Burn out can happen in any profession, but it's especially devastating to an actor because their whole career is built on faith. If I do this and this, I will get here. The fact is that many actors do the right things and never get the rewards they think they deserve. The body and mind can only take so much rejection and battle fatigue before it waves the white flag. Sometimes, this might not be a bad thing.

If you are burnt out, then maybe it's time to stop fighting it. You don't need to quit the business, maybe you just need to take a break. Many actors have taken a sabbatical and return to the business some years later to achieve far more success than they had had previously.

Refocusing, reenergizing, stepping away, and regaining perspective can give a burnt-out actor a fresh start. Now, I am not a psychologist (nor have I yet played one on television), but if your problem is deeper than that, you might consider speaking to someone professionally. Long-term depression is usually more than a career issue and goes beyond this kind of career burn out.

Then there is the complete burn out. There are some tremendously gifted actors who are no longer in the business because they reached that very point. They are not coming back to the fold.

If you find yourself at that place, please don't look at it as failure. It's growth into new areas for you. You've accomplished so much already. You were a professional actor and you'll always have that. You did what you loved and you gave it your all. There is absolutely nothing wrong with turning your attentions to new passions, fresh adventures, and a whole new career if you choose. It's not about how far you get as an actor, it's that you did it and how you did it. Life is just too short to keep doing something if it no longer makes you happy.

C

Casting Directors

No group will likely have so much effect on your professional life as will casting directors. Casting directors, or CDs as actors often call them, can be your best ally, or they can be an unsolvable puzzle. Those two types—one who brings you in regularly and one whom you'll never meet—might be just a door away from each other in the same building. In Los Angeles, there are hundreds of them casting films, television programs, commercials, voice-overs, music videos, theatre, print ads, and so on, and yet thousands of actors cry the all too familiar refrain, "I can't get an audition!"

Walk into any one of the multitude of caster's offices throughout the metropolitan area and you'll quickly learn why. There are pictures everywhere; pictures are covering the desks and piled on the floors, the cabinets, the furniture, and any other available open space. There are even pictures on the walls, and that's where you want to be because those shots are usually the people who've just been cast in a project.

With so many actors sending pictures for relatively few roles, it's amazing anyone ever gets any auditions, but they do and so will you if you market consistently, build relationships and keep your skills at a high level.

It works pretty much like this. A casting director is hired by a producer, studio, or network to put together the acting ensemble for a show. The caster may be a full-time employee, which is often the case when one has established herself by putting together the casts of hit programs.

However, many top casting directors are independents. They sort of operate like actors—working job to job, show to show, and sooner or later looking for their next gig. Let's face it, not every show is a "Seinfeld" that lasts for years making everyone involved, including the casters, stars.

Whatever a casting director's status—employee or freelancer—if they've ever cast one legitimate project, their offices will be filled with 8×10s of actors young and old aching to read for them. In the past, there was something called *"generals,"* which meant actors would actually get a chance to sit in front of a casting director at an informal meeting. This was not an audition per se, just a face to face to see what the actor was about so that the caster could potentially place them for future role readings.

Generals have gone the way of the Movie of the Week. They hardly exist anymore. They may happen once in a blue moon, but no one expects to meet a casting director in that fashion today. The best way you're going to see one today is through your own consistent marketing, your agent doing his job, and probably a continued combination of both of those things.

It is often said in Hollywood that casting directors have long memories and might bring an actor back long after he has met them, sometime even after years. Possible, if you're wonderful, but don't count on it. You want to get cast when you are in front of the people. This business is too tough to let any opportunity slip by for hope of another day. To help that process, you want to make sure you consistently nail auditions and establish as many quality casting contacts as possible and hope *some* of them, who can't use you right now, will remember you for future opportunities.

Two things can happen when you read for a CD. You'll either do well enough to get a callback (always preferable) or you won't (happens to the best of them). If you don't get that follow-up audition, two more things could happen. You may never read for the person again, or they might keep your picture for another gig later down the line. They'll only do that if you are good, even if you weren't right for the role for which you just read. That's something a surviving actor must think about. You must be prepared and well rehearsed before you read for someone, even if you end up being wrong for a particular role, because not only are you reading for that particular part, you are showcasing your acting skills for all future casting possibilities.

Casting is a subjective business. What one casting director likes, the other might not. You won't get every job. You probably won't get most of them. Although you'll never be able to please everyone, you are still obligated as a professional actor to go in for each call fully prepared. Survivors prepare. Successful actors prepare even more. Others wing it.

Talk with any casting director in Hollywood, and they'll all mention the actors who don't take advantage of their audition opportunities.

Caster Lisa Miller Katz succinctly notes, "It happens all the time, and if someone is not prepared, I can see it almost immediately. If they're unprepared and I can tell, they probably will never get there, I thank them and that's that."

Richard Hicks, who has cast many features including "Igby Goes Down" and "Hope Floats" as well as the HBO series "Curb Your Enthusiasm," concurs on the preparedness factor:

> The actor who gets the role is the one who prepares—the one who has invested a lot of himself in this. Most people come in and they do a nice job. They do a perfectly acceptable job, but they don't do an amazing job. So make a pact with yourself not to waste those opportunities.

To survive in Hollywood and the process of casting, you should also accept this simple fact: You will never meet all the casting directors. It doesn't happen, no matter how good you are. If you've come from a smaller market, you've probably known and read for all four or five of the CDs that held the keys to the good jobs. In Los Angeles, you have four or five on the same floor in the same office building, and there are a lot of floors and buildings in this city. The number of casting directors combined with associates and assistants is staggering. Although you'll never be able to meet them all, that doesn't mean you don't give it your best shot. Be a solid performer and a busy marketer as well.

Market yourself to casters, market some more, and then do it again. When you finally get an agent, you still market. You'll burn through thousands of postcards and headshots over time, but after dozens of mailings it takes only one amazing audition for a casting director to make it all worth your while.

Most CDs love actors and are in their corner—no surprise, given that they spend much of their days with them. Many casters were, and in some cases still are, actors. They want you to do well and will often help you to get there. They bring in new faces all the time and are loyal to the old faces who've worked for them before. They'll go to bat for you when they think you're right for the role, even if their boss is looking in another direction. That's as good as it gets for an actor. All right, maybe that followed by a booking is slightly better.

However, there are some CDs who can frustrate actors. A few are known to favor performers only from certain agencies. A few are snobbish and unprofessional. A few are known to not even particularly like actors much. As actors, we tend to put casting directors on a pedestal because they have so much to do with our success or lack thereof. Respect the person, not the image of the person, and all in all, you'll have many more positive experiences with these professionals than negative ones throughout the years.

Over time, you'll establish a series of relationships and probably find that you've gotten on the short list of small number of casters who know you, and bring you in from time to time. Those cherished relationships can be the foundation for your Los Angeles acting career.

Casting Director Workshops

Nothing in the last few years has generated as much debate amongst Los Angeles actors as have casting director workshops. The workshops are run by a variety of independent companies who pay casters, and occasionally agents, to come in and watch scenes and perhaps critique actors' performances.

The fact that casters are being paid for their presence isn't a problem for many people, it's who has to pay to see them—actors. Therein lies the problem. Whether you're for or against this method of meeting industry hirers, the fact is that casting workshops require actors to essentially buy the right to audition for the potential of future work. That point has engendered a lot of passion on both sides, and the CD workshop arena now under the microscope may be changing in one way or another in the future.

What was once a small sideline to meet a handful of industry people has now become big business. The days of general meetings, whereby casters met new actors in their offices has pretty much disappeared. Many actors feel generals have been replaced with this paid form of being seen. It's not a pretty picture and the battle lines are growing stronger each day on this matter.

Actors who attend workshops praise them as a great resource for getting seen by casting directors they are unable to normally meet. The happiest performers are those who have actually gotten hired for paid acting work later by the same casters. The most vociferous supporters claim no one has the right to tell them how and, in this case, how much they should be paying to meet someone that might help their careers. Another group that does workshops but can't get that excited claim they are a necessary evil. One actor wrote me and said, "If I don't do them I have no shot at all." Actors who are against them say they are ruining the integrity of the caster–actor relationships.

Detractors claim workshops are a huge conflict of interest. They say, no actor should have to pay anyone for a meeting. CDs and agents already earn money, why should they make actors pay to be seen? Workshop devotees have no problem with meeting and reading for casting personnel this way, even if it costs them some money.

Here's how they work. The workshops are almost all cold reading—an actor gets the sides, has a few minutes or more to work with a partner, and then does the scene for whoever the industry guest is that evening. Sometimes it's a working CD, and sometimes it's an assistant from the office. They'll tell you a little about what they cast and then it's right into the readings. The paid guests will either critique the scenes or remain passive observers. When the performances are done, they'll collect headshots and be on their way. Whether they ever bring an actor in for a real audition during business hours is the big gamble that many actors are willing to pay for.

Actors have often written to the "Tombudsman" column querying on my opinion. I don't do the workshops and personally won't pay to meet anyone, but I am also aware that they have been beneficial to a number of actors hoping to meet someone who might hire them. That *number* is of great debate between the pro- and anti-workshop sides.

Still, the bottom line is, should an actor have to resort to this type of paid showcase to meet industry people in the first place? Is it ethical for a casting director, who already has a job, to even ask performers to pony $20 or $30 for the right to read a scene? When pressed, most actors will tell you they aren't happy that they have to pay, and this comes from some who participate in the workshops.

Meanwhile, everyone is afraid to complain for fear they'll insult someone, rock the boat, or perhaps invite litigation. The Casting Society of America remains mum. ATA doesn't make a peep, and SAG is very careful about condemning anything that might put them in an awkward position regarding their friends the casting directors. Not surprisingly, most actors share their opinions with only those they trust.

How many casters participate in these cold reading workshops? Nowhere near the majority, but enough, and some who cast major projects, so you can see why actors are drawn to them like a moth to the flame.

So the debate rages on. By the looks of things it'll continue that way, although as this book was being published, the issue was finally being put to the legal test due to a vociferous opposition campaign against workshops started some time ago by an organization called DoNot-Pay.org.

Due to this group's relentless crusade against workshops, the California Department of Labor Standards Enforcement issued an opinion on January 22, 2002, stating that "casting director cold reading workshops constitute a clear violation of the provisions of section 450 of the California Labor Code." In February, the agency had just begun mailing cease and desist letters to owners of many of the workshops, although it's been made clear that casting directors who participate in the classes will not be targeted in any legal actions that might occur.

This legal step will certainly stoke the fires of this issue and may lead to the end of workshops as they exist today. However, the workshop owners are a formidable force and will undoubtedly not go down without a fight. They are currently circling the wagons, and a lengthy battle is sure to be in the works. In July 2002, many workshops continue, claiming their enterprise is an educational environment and therefore is completely legal. Actors will be watching closely.

Cold Reading

If you're auditioning for television, then sooner or later you are going to be cold reading. Cold reading can be defined as someone handing you sides at the audition, giving you just a few minutes to look them over, and bringing you into the audition room to read.

This happens on occasion in television when hot off the computer rewrites are substituted for old sides, but true cold reads are usually reserved for commercial auditions. There they usually present little problem because many commercials today are light on copy and big on visuals.

You'll find ample classes and discussion on the subject of cold reading, but the truth is you won't be doing all that much actual cold reading in audition situations. Nevertheless, the preparation in getting you to work with new sides, understanding the scene, and building a character quickly will help you in any audition situation.

For film auditions, you'll often have your material several days in advance. Call these hot reads and you better hope you are hot, too, because good film auditions are hard to snag. In television, where you'll likely have more opportunities, you should have your sides at least a full day in advance to work on them, so you might consider these reads warm ones rather than cold.

Whether given a week, a day, or less than an hour—a surviving actor must polish a performance to a professional level or he doesn't survive for long. Mastering cold reading for those last-minute script change scenarios can make the difference between booking the job or spending another day unemployed.

In those true cold situations when you get new material at the last minute, you cannot freak out. Sometimes you might even be the only actor in the waiting room who is still holding old material. Buckle down and get to work on the new stuff, but don't overly concern yourself with memorizing under such pressure. Get the first two lines in your head and the last one or two, and then use the material during the audition. Remember, the producers want you to be good, and part of being good is saying the lines that someone took the trouble to write for you, even if you've just gotten them. That training will come in handy during these situations. It's also not uncommon to have them ask you to read for another role, and this is a very nice cold reading scenario because it means they like your work and are trying to find a role for you.

However, in most cases, you will be working on one character with material previously furnished. Naturally, the responsibility is on you to get your audition material as soon as possible and to work on it enough so that you are in character and nearly off-book (memorized) by the time you show up. Given the proliferation of Internet sites where you can download your sides immediately upon getting an audition call (Showfax and Castnet are the two big competitors offering this service), there is usually no reason to be cold in that room. You would think no one would arrive unprepared, yet from conversations I've had with casting directors, it apparently happens enough of the time to bear repeating. You're a professional. Work on the material. The person who gets the job does.

Commercial Auditioning

Talk about cattle calls. You could go to a hundred film or television show casting sessions and never see the number of actors that you'd encounter in one week of commercial auditions. Commercial casters either rent huge rehearsal spaces for auditions or, if they're really successful, have their own full-time facilities to handle these sometimes outrageously large gatherings. An actor might show up at a large facility and see only a few names on a sign-in sheet. He soon realizes he's only looking at page one of twelve that have yet to be filled with two day's worth of talent.

The American commercial industry spends well over $30 billion each year in pursuit of trying to sell you something you probably don't need. They succeed brilliantly. Some of that money can end up in the hands of working actors, and how long you are willing to take on the mission of pursuing the elusive magic spot might determine your chances for success here. Acting might be a numbers game to some degree, but commercial acting is a numbers game times a numbers game. To get a commercial, you have to find the proverbial needle in the haystack. Getting an acting job after dozens of auditions might seem like a huge victory until you understand the remuneration isn't what you thought it would be.

Although commercial employment can still mean big monetary rewards, although nothing like the halcyon days of the past, the process of getting that work can be demoralizing and taxing to even the strongest of the lot. Many actors avoid commercials altogether and stick to the arenas of film, television, and theatre, where they believe there is some reasonable chance for landing work. How's that for a novelty—film, television and theatre being considered *easier* to get?

Most of the time you'll be competing for these jobs with others like yourself—professional actors. Some spots, however, might just seek the right face, actor or otherwise, and this is where you find the amateurs flooding in. This irks professional actors, one whom quipped at a commercial audition, filled with actors auditioning for the role of car salesmen alongside real car salesmen, "You don't see us at their dealership trying to sell a car, do you?"

Many of the better commercials offer meaty roles, almost minifilms, which require the talents of only the strongest of actors. Whatever the role, they'll be plenty of bodies lining up for a chance to pitch a product.

Caster Jacob Ferret, of the very hip and busy Funky Ferrets Casting, duly notes, "If there is a Breakdown out for one character in a spot, we get anywhere from five-hundred to one thousand submissions per character."

Gulp.

Fellow Ferret, Robert, adds,

> In commercials, it's a huge numbers game. How many pictures we get depends on the character. If we're casting for a kid, there's going to be a lot more submissions than if we were casting for a seventy-year old man. If we're casting females 30–35, very natural, very real that means three thousand.

Double gulp.

Commercials are obviously of major interest to actors and their talent representatives. Why? It's acting work, and it's sometimes very highly paid acting work. Between a good session and a healthy ad run, an actor could make more income in one year from a single day of work on a commercial than he would over a lifetime from a television show or film's residuals. In fact, more income from sessions and residuals is derived from commercials than from either film or television jobs. The year 2000 was an exception due to a lengthy commercial strike.

Commercials are also more receptive to considering less experienced actors breaking in here. In fact, it's a respectable entry into SAG for many younger, nonunion performers.

Agent Patty Grana-Miller explains, "While it would be very difficult without your SAG card to be represented in the theatrical arena, in commercials some agents will certainly consider nonunion performers because it's much easier to Taft–Hartley you."

Taft–Hartley allows a nonunion actor or even a nonactor to work for up to thirty days on union projects. You'll be paid and treated as a union actor. If you're done in two days, you have another twenty-eight days to seek other union gigs without becoming a member. You can also still do nonunion jobs. After the thirty-day period and when you are offered another union job, you must then join SAG.

Robert Ferret concurs. "Commercials are always an easier way to break in versus the theatrical side," adds Ferret. "It's because a lot of times commercials are just based on look."

Of the big paydays of commercials past, he notes,

Up until the early 90's you could book one national commercial and
you were set for the year. Now if you book twelve commercials you
still haven't made the same amount of money as you would have
on that one. You do a national spot now and there's no telling if it
is going to run period. Usually ad agencies hold off for two or three
airing cycles and then run it. If it gets a negative response that puppy is
gone, no matter how much money they spent on the campaign. Then
again there are still products out there that run for the full twenty-one
months and they do renegotiations.

When that happens, and it's all too rare, actors have hit the jackpot.
More often though, a commercial airs for perhaps a cycle (thirteen
weeks) or two and then disappears into the abyss. They are hardly the
ticket to financial freedom they once were or were believed to be, yet
actors still seek them out like they were the Holy Grail.

It isn't easy. Just listen to Jeff Gerrard who casts many major spots
at his Big House Studios in Universal City:

I know a lot of actors that have been discouraged just the way the
whole system has changed and because of the enormous amount of
actors that have come into the business. Years ago you used to have
five people for the total callback. Nowadays you have maybe twenty-
five on callback for each role.

The bottom line: You could go to several dozen commercial calls
and never get a single job. That would likely mean the end to a career for a television or film actor but in commercials it's the norm.
Eventually though, to succeed, you'll need to get some results and that
usually starts with callbacks, being invited back for the follow-up audition where you'll meet the director and creative team behind the
commercial. Regardless of whether you get the gig, consistently getting
callbacks is a strong indicator that you're doing something very right
and are a marketable commercial type. It'll probably only be a matter
of time before you get your first booking.

Who is getting the work in this new millennium? Well, there is
still a preponderance of the physically beautiful in commercials, but
nowadays pretty much all types are seen pitching in commercials.

Gerrard observes,

When I first started twenty years ago it was basically if you're blonde-
haired and blue-eyed and you can walk and talk and you have a
great smile and your teeth were straight you were definitely booking
between $25,000 and $100,000 a year. Nowadays it's very much the
real person. It's the average person on the street and it's a very real
texture that many directors are looking for.

The auditions are run fairly similarly, regardless of where they take place. You show up, face a room full of eager beavers, sign in, and fill out a size sheet—just in case you book the darn thing. Someone appears from behind a door, takes a Polaroid of you, and then you wait your turn. While waiting, you look at the audition material and try to think of how you're going to make an impression to separate yourself from the masses.

In film and television, it's you, the caster, and maybe a reader, but in commercials you'll need to factor in that you're not only auditioning but you're often also doing so with other performers. Don't look at them as competition, although they very well may be, look at them as part of your ensemble. Generally, but not always, if you work together, the entire crew might get a callback. If one actor tries to dominate the proceedings, it can sabotage it for everybody. Do your best acting and respect that you are there with other players. Get a bit in, do your part to stand out (it might just be a great look), and then support the rest of your team. It'll work better for you in the long run.

When they call you in, you state your name on-camera, some ask you to strangely turn from side to side, as in a mug-shot scenario, and you read the copy. If there is copy. Assuming there is actually something to read, they almost always have cue cards at commercial sessions. There's the help I was talking about. That's something you'd never find at a reading for a television show or film, and they always put you on tape, which happens only rarely for television and film.

Commercial actor Richard Ransbottom, who has done spots for I-Hop and 7-Up, offers this on the difference between a commercial and film audition:

> They're very different. Commercials are much freer and quicker, and by that I mean they're running you through, where as on a theatrical call they'll normally spend a little more time with you and try to work with you. I've gone in on commercials and they've had no script. They just start asking you a bunch of questions. You're supposed to be witty and show what you can do.

Actress Marla Martenson has been in the same boat enough times to speak knowingly on the subject:

> You have to stand out. You have to do something to hook their atten-tion. It's always good to have a little story because it's often improv, and they'll ask you something like, "What was your most embarrass-ing moment?" or "What was your funniest date?" I found that's when I always got the job, when I had them laughing.

When improvisation isn't involved you'll work from the script, which is not held in your hand as it would be at a television audition, but is on a cue card alongside the camera. If you're going to try commercial work, get some training in working with cue cards. They can be very disconcerting to an actor coming from theatre and even film work.

Commercial actors do something you'd hardly ever see at an audition for film or television shows. They dress up for the part. I don't mean a suit and tie, although that may very well be the outfit appropriate for the part. If you go to a call for policemen, most of the actors there will be dressed in cop uniforms. If the part is for a waitress, you can be sure many of the actresses will have something like a skirt, an apron, and probably a pencil behind their ear. Some actors scoff at this, but then see the actors dressed like cowboys, doctors, and nurses. Finally, they catch on and do the same thing. Other actors don't go for that approach, but try to suggest the role in their appearance. A construction worker for one actor might mean a tool belt, helmet, and a bandana but to another a dusty t-shirt and jeans. There's no right way. Whatever works for you. The actors that do dress the role full tilt think their chances are better because the tape is shipped back to the client who looks at the tape and makes their cuts. It stands to reason that if there are two equally talented actors up for a role and one looks more like the part, he might get the role more often.

One other aspect of commercial auditioning differs from film and television reads. In commercial reads, you will often be working with other actors on-camera. Many spots have multiple characters, and it's not uncommon for two, three, or five actors to audition together. You might be reading for a pit crew or a group of high school students on their way to the prom. As such, the energy level can be quite high.

After the auditions are completed, the tapes are sent to the ad agency in charge of the campaign, the client, who pays the ad agency, and the director, all of whom make the choices of whom they'll bring in again for the callback. With so many people making picks, the numbers can be high the next time around. One actor I know, sourly calls them . . . the *all* backs.

Unlike the first audition, at the callback, usually held a few days after the first call, the director will be in attendance, the ad agency people will be there, and many times the client will show up as well. Talk about scaling Mt. Everest. Now you've got to impress a roomful of very opinionated people, who often don't see eye to eye on who should get the gig. Usually—and this shouldn't surprise you—the client, who controls the purse strings, makes the ultimate choice when the parties in attendance aren't in full agreement on who should be cast.

Robert Ferret explains, "When it comes to the callback, and you're in that situation, a lot of times you could be the best actor but you might not get the role. It's all bureaucratic. It's all show business and there's much more business than there is show."

Commissions

Commissions require only two things, understanding them and paying them to your agent and/or manager. They actually work rather simply until you start digging through the layers and then like everything else they gain complexity. In the union world, it's fairly basic. If you are paid above union scale for AFTRA or SAG work, you'll be required to pay your agent ten percent of your gross earnings. If you're paid scale, then an automatic ten percent will be on top of the fee as set by union minimum requirements. In other words, the producer pays your agent the commission, not you.

When you are responsible for the fee, much of the time you won't have to worry about cutting a check because your agent will have previously required you to sign a check authorization form allowing them to get your paycheck directly from the employer. They then snip off their ten percent from the top before forwarding you the remaining balance.

However, on rare occasions an agented actor will still find the original check arriving at their home instead of their agent's office. If this happens, do exactly what your agent does. Make a copy of the check and then deposit it in your bank account, and just as soon as it clears you'll cut a check for ten percent of the gross, and get it to your rep.

If on occasion you've found your agency doesn't forward the checks to you as quickly as they should, this is not an opportunity for revenge. Do the right thing and forward the fee immediately upon clearance in your account. No exceptions. Lead by example even if your agency hasn't necessarily warranted such a demonstration.

If you have a manager, you're more than likely going to owe them fifteen percent. It can be more for nonunion people, so check the contract closely before signing, although I suggest you steer clear of anyone charging much more.

From that original gross payment, write yet another check for fifteen percent and send it off with a copy of the check and pay statement to your manager. When all your commissions, minus Uncle Sam's hefty cut, are removed from your check, it'll seem that everyone got paid but you. Have no fear. At tax time, you'll deduct those commissions paid and get some of it back.

Now let's talk about the lifeline of the surviving actor known as residuals. It's pretty cut and dry here as well. In most cases, if a residual commission is due to your agent, the union will mail you a little slip telling you they've sent a payment to your agency. (Note: Recent changes are redefining what is commissionable and what is not, rerunwise. Check with SAG or AFTRA if you have any questions.)

If you haven't gotten your payment from your agency within ten days or so of them having received it, it's time to call your agency's accounting department. Their reply will usually be, "We just put it in the mail."

Quite often a film or television residual check will come directly to you from the union. In most instances when it arrives directly, you are not required to pay a commission. However, with all the changes in the air, there are sure to be some mistakes in the next couple of years. Upon signing your agency contract, make sure they spell out what is commissionable. Double check this information with the union and guild, and you'll be properly advised.

In the commercial world, everything is commissionable. If you get paid, your agent gets paid. If you get the check, do the right thing and pay the appropriate commission to your agent. If you run into any problems with commissions and you're a union person, call the appropriate office and they'll spell out the right way to handle these money issues.

What if you're nonunion? If you're working with an agency that is franchised by SAG or AFTRA, you'll be treated pretty much the same as a union actor and receive timely payments. If however, you're nonunion and working with one of the licensed (as agencies are required by California law) nonfranchised agencies, you're usually going to be waiting longer for your money.

It commonly takes nonunion actors thirty or more days to get their payments for jobs, but they can find the wait is just starting once their talent representative has gotten the check. Suffice it to say, work only with an agency or management company that treats you as they would a union client. You'll rarely, if ever, receive your money as quickly as a union actor would (usually a couple of weeks) but if you're commonly finding delays of six weeks or more, and you know your rep has gotten your payment sent to them, then you either have to lay down the law or move on to a new agency.

Nonunion actors become super sleuths. If they feel they're being taken advantage of, they sometimes call the producer directly to see if the payment has been made. If it has, the producer is usually as upset about the money not being put into the hands of the talent in a reasonable timeframe, as is the actor. I've heard from a few performers who did this, the producer called the talent rep and the money miraculously was paid to the actor within a couple of days.

Your agency, franchised or not, should operate professionally so that it never comes to that. If you have a quality talent representative, you'll get paid without hassle most of the time.

The process is much the same as for a union actor. You'll receive a check that has the commission deducted from the gross, although commission charges are commonly higher for nonunion actors. Quite often the fee is twenty percent. A few attempt to charge even more. In my opinion, anything higher than twenty percent is a genuine rip-off and should be avoided. A small number of nonfranchised agents only charge clients the same ten percent as would be found in the franchised world. Good luck finding one of them.

It's not uncommon for a nonunion performer's agent to add a twenty percent fee on top of your gross when billing the producer. You might ask yourself, why should you have to pay any commission if the agent is already billing the producer a charge of an additional twenty percent? That's an excellent question that you can debate over for years. Double-dipping is very commonplace in the nonunion world. You either accept it or seek out a different representative who will contractually agree to not take a commission from you if the producer pays them a fee on top of what you are making. Can an actor dare demand not paying a commission when they've already gotten it from a producer? Most actors can't, but if you're a consistent booker and highly popular client with casting directors, you may be able to work a deal that's more along the lines of a union actor. Contracts can be amended a hundred different ways to suit each professional relationship. You didn't really think stars were paying their agents' ten percent did you?

Managers usually get fifteen percent from nonunion thespians. Rarely would they be paid by the producer, as the agent usually negotiates the contract. I say *usually* because on occasion managers do the negotiation, even though they aren't legally supposed to, and if that's the case you might find them getting the aforementioned double-dip commission fee. Ask them and they'll either tell you or they won't, but you can dig up the information and use it to negotiate a better contract.

If you manage to miraculously get the original check sent directly by the producer, upon clearance, pay all your talent representatives what your contract says you're supposed to pay. Never, and I repeat, never, fail to pay your proper commissions, even if you are leaving an agency or manager. Only end professional relationships when the slate is clean on all moneys due.

If you've been stiffed and it's been more than a couple of months and you've made calls and still aren't getting paid for a nonunion project, call the Department of Consumer Affairs to seek information on your legal rights.

Consistency

The truth is there are lots of good actors who could be great actors, but many never get that chance. You need to work a lot to develop into the next level of performer. It's not just a gift you're born with. You have to use it regularly and improve upon it.

It's all about consistency and that only comes from hanging in long enough to build a steady work schedule. Consistency by average working actor standards might mean getting a real gig every month or every six months. You're at the mercy of the people who hire but you can't let that stop you. Ideally, you'll get enough on-set acting work to keep you semi-employed and growing as an actor. You'll consistently and slowly build to higher and higher levels. Maybe a few actors truly are born with extraordinary talent, but most learn it and build upon it by daily acting work of some type.

So what do you do if the phone isn't ringing for auditions? You go to class. How about if you can't even afford to go to class this month? You improvise. Maybe literally. You work on acting in your living room, in your dining room, on your roof—if it's not slanted. You read lines opposite your roommate or your cat. You go through scripts and break down characters. You do voice work in your car. You observe free theatre, meet informally with other actors, watch film and television closely, hang at a performance arts bookstore, something—anything other than avoiding it because it's easier. There is opportunity to improve your abilities everywhere, every day if you choose, but you have to take the first step.

Otherwise, you become too reliant on getting a job to improve your skills and that's not the way to approach this thing. The job is really the bonus that arrives gift wrapped every once in awhile.

When actual work comes, the preparation you did on your own will make it all the better. If you do something every day you get better at it, whether you're in front of the camera, in front of a classroom, or in front of your couch. It's a consistent approach to your career. It comes back to you in a big way.

Continuity

You're hired as an actor primarily to do a great job portraying a character, but they've also hired you, the pro, for another reason—to be smart. Part of that is to help protect the integrity of the project. You do this by understanding continuity and being a keen observer of your own performance.

There is a wonderful person on set known as the script supervisor. Making sure the director has every shot he needs is her primary objective, but she is there for you for two other reasons. During rehearsal and shooting, she'll feed you a line if you require assistance, but most important, she'll watch over you so that you don't screw up on the continuity. For example, "You reached for the beer with your left hand on that line," that kind of stuff.

Script supervisors are usually there to help, but you are ultimately responsible for your own continuity issues. They've got a lot of people to watch. You only have one. Surviving actors learn to cover themselves.

It really can amount to a survival issue—whether you'll survive getting cut. I'm assuming you want to end up in the final edit. You can help make that happen by not causing an amateurish mistake in regard to matching what you held, wore, or even smoked during the previous shots. Yes, there are ways directors can cut around a continuity flub ("we'll fix it in post" is the common refrain), but don't count on it. Sometimes they'll just cut your coverage or even the whole scene if they can't cover it.

A continuity example: You're playing a cop. As they shoot the master, on each take you pull your gun out on a particular line and put it back in the holster on another. Six hours later, when they get around to shooting the scene from another angle, are you going to remember exactly when you pulled the gun, how high you held it, whether you had your finger on the trigger, and whether you held it head high, chest high, and so on?

Be aware of what you do. Don't create too much business for yourself that will only potentially hinder you in the end. Anytime you're using a prop, the continuity error factor rises. If it's a prop that changes sizes (cigars, glass of soda pop), be triply aware. Nothing looks sillier than seeing a full cigar in a master and then a stub of one in a close-up a moment later.

A smart actor learns to be his own continuity supervisor. He also makes a friend he'll probably never meet on the set—the film editor.

Coverage

Coverage is something working actors have a keen knowledge of. It is the manner in which the director and his cinematographer film the action of a scene. In simple terms, it's a master shot that involves moving the camera in closer to the actors at whatever angles and frame sizes they deem necessary to convey the artistic and emotional palette they're trying to convey. There are as many ways to cover a scene as there are ideas in the director's head.

To a surviving actor, the coverage issue usually reflects how much time you are ultimately going to get to define your part.

The general rule of thumb is the smaller the part the less coverage you'll get and, therefore, the less takes. Be ready for that and if it gets any better be very appreciative for the time and opportunity devoted to your contribution to the entire scene. As a visiting actor, you can usually count on being part of the master and maybe one angle—probably a medium shot of you talking to the other actor. They'll save the high-impact close-ups, in most cases anyway, for the stars and guest stars.

Let's say you're a day player, the usual actor hired for one or two days in a smaller principal role. You'll be around the set for many hours, witnessing countless hours designated to lighting and filming the star or series regulars with whom you may be doing your scene. That makes sense—the show is about them and their storyline after all. It may be hours of various lighting and filming schemes devoted to making your fellow actor look their best. If it's a film, it may be a full day!

For the sake of this scenario, let's pop you in the scene with the name actor because it stands a much better chance of getting you something beyond a wide master, which they'd often do with a cast of unknowns.

So you do the master shot once or twice and then they light for the star's angles. Naturally, there's plenty of time here. You'll stand next to the camera and do your lines so that you can make eye contact and assist the star while they shoot her.

Then, sooner or later, they'll turn the camera around and point it at you. Don't be alarmed if the pace suddenly picks up or you hear the director saying to the cameraman something such as, "We'll just grab a quick shot of him." It's not a reflection of you; that's just the way it's done in Hollywood.

You'll probably get a medium shot with two or three takes. If you don't nail it, they'll probably live with it as they don't want to spend too much time on day players or sometimes even on guest stars. That's ultimately the key to what you need to know on coverage—you won't get a lot of it until you're a big time star. Make the most of any shot you're in because you won't have a lot of time or film on which to improve it further.

Crashing Auditions

Sooner or later, nearly every actor ponders the question of whether to crash an audition. There is one type of crashing in which anyone of good sense would never partake. Do not deceive a casting office into thinking you are supposed to be there for an audition time that wasn't scheduled. When someone tries to sneak in by adding their name to a sign-in sheet, they are setting themselves up for a rude awakening. They almost always get caught and may never be invited to that office again.

Improperly signing is different than merely arriving at the right place at the right time with picture in hand. That's tricky in and of itself because each casting office has its own tolerance level about people dropping by.

Now there are ways to crash without breaking the rules. A well-timed picture drop might actually be prudent as long as you don't overuse the system. Let's say you become aware of a role for which you are perfect. They're looking for an actor 6'5", 280 pounds, who has experience as a poker dealer. What if that's you to a "T"? As a surviving actor, you'd be making a big mistake if you didn't do something to get in front of them for that role. If your agent hasn't been able to get you an appointment, you should do some marketing and drop a headshot/resume at the office—assuming they allow drop-offs—before the role is cast.

Respect that there's business going on and get out of their way. A picture drop-off shouldn't take more than a minute; if you hang around much longer, you're probably doing yourself more harm than good.

The proper way is to bring in the picture and give it to the person at the front desk. If that's not acceptable, drop it into the box for the appropriate show. You could certainty leave a note on the picture saying you are submitting for the role of X on the television show. Because they are casting the show in timely fashion, you increase your chances of actually getting an audition. If you drop the picture off on the actual date they are holding a call, you might hit the lottery and be given a chance to audition. It's a very slim chance, but it happens on occasion. Never stop the casting director or interrupt a casting session by asking if you can audition? In film and TV casting, they will not allow you to do so.

In commercials, there are many more crashers than there are in the film world. Due to large numbers of actors who read for spots, it is not unheard of for an actor to squeeze into the audition, sign in, and actually get an unscheduled audition. I promise you this. Do it and you might get away with it once or twice, even if they're reading hundreds of actors, but you will eventually get caught and piss someone off. Do you really want to do that? Is one job worth it?

Commercial casting directors, the Funky Ferrets, explain, "You don't want to crash. Crashing is definitely against the rules. There are people that we have caught trying to crash and they've said they had a scheduled appointment. We found out they didn't and we had to turn them away." But the Ferrets are quick to explain that trying to deceive and just being aggressive are very different:

> We've had actors who have just shown up to casting and asked, "Hey, am I right for this?" And on occasion we've gone, "Absolutely, you're right, sign in," and they've ended up booking the job. There have also been actors who have asked that and we've said, "No, you're not right." Both of those situations, however, are different than someone signing in and acting as if they already had an appointment. That's crashing and it's wrong.

Quite different is the appropriately dropped off picture. If you get good information that a commercial is being cast, no one will hate you for dropping a headshot to the right box. This is different than signing in and trying to act as if you have an appointment.

Not long ago, I heard about a role I was just right for in a big commercial. My plan was simple, I knew they were casting all week, so on the previous Friday I put together a picture and resume for an early Monday drop-off. On Monday I stopped by the office, double-parked, because I knew I'd be in and out in thirty seconds, and I ran into the office to drop my picture into the appropriate caster's box, which I knew was right inside the main door. I leaned over to put my picture in the already overflowing box when a young woman said, "I'll take that." "Thank you," I said. I turned to walk out to my car and she stopped me. "You're perfect for this. You can stay and read now if you'd like."

D

Demo Reels

In Hollywood, a resume is great, but a demo reel is even better. Being in this visual medium, agents, casting directors, producers, and directors often like to see their prospective charges in action. Naturally an audition is the ultimate way to make that happen, but a demo can open the door for you and perhaps keep it open should it come down to two or three actors for a part.

Do you have a demo? Do you have a reel? Do you have a copy of your work? These are questions you'll hear all the time. You'll want to be able to answer, "Yes."

Demo reels are visual clips from your work, preferably professional ones from film, television, commercials, maybe industrials, and occasionally theatre that are cut into a nicely edited two- to seven-minute video presentations. They are primarily used to attract the attention of talent agents. However, hirers also view them regularly, particularly when casting for show leads or if they can't make a decision on some equally qualified performers. A persuasive agent can even sway someone to view your demo in consideration for future parts.

Talent agent Craig Wyckoff, of Epstein-Wyckoff, Corsa, Ross offers to explain the significance of the demo in this market:

> They're very important. It's good for getting an agent, because there is nothing we hate worse than seeing a scene in the office. It's an artificial environment and it's really hard for actors to do a good job in the office. When you view a demo you're looking to see if the work is good, is the actor marketable, and do I go, "Wow!" Because if I go "Wow," then when I send it to a casting director they're going to go "Wow" as well. We send tapes to everyone—studio and network people, executives, producers. When you are making your demo, be very honest with yourself and say, based on this, would I hire me?

There are no shortages of businesses that will cut together your demo tape. You won't need to spend more than a couple hundred dollars to have a serviceable reel, maybe twice that amount for a superior one.

Your best clips, and preferably those from recent shows, should come first. A well-regarded theory is that directors watch about thirty seconds of these things before they scan search the rest or hit the stop button. So if you can wow 'em in the first thirty seconds, they may not touch the scan button.

A beginning actor won't have much material for a reel, but this is no reason to rush out and put fake scenes or single camera long-shot selections from a stage play you did in the past. A professional demo doesn't have classroom scenes, high school plays, or monologues. It's stuff you would see on television and in films. Busier professional actors sometimes even have two demos—one of theatrical clips (film/TV) and another of commercial work. It's a very vital tool in today's market.

However, no one expects a youngish newcomer to already have a demo. If you are a young and marketable type, agents will still see you. Casting directors will still read you. Hollywood adores youth. A great headshot and some regional credits will do fine to start you off.

It's not quite as easy if you're in your thirties or forties. At this juncture, they expect you to have clips of your work. If you don't, you'd better get real busy trying to land independent or student films, to build a starter reel.

In the day-to-day business of casting costars and guest roles, much of that work is done without a reel ever being requested or seen. A Breakdown is released, actors' headshots or names are submitted, and some of them get appointments. So for practical purposes, consider your demo reel as part of the bigger picture. It's good to have one as soon as you can, but don't rush something unprofessional into the marketplace.

Once you've eventually booked two or three professional parts, take those clips into a demo editor and start the editing process. You'll usually supply the masters, which you can often get from the production company you've worked for, and you'll view the different clips available to use. It's always better to get a master as there is less image degradation.

Video Editor Sharon Stephens suggests these basics when you're planning your reel:

> Your demo should project the image as to how you want to be seen by casting directors, producers and directors. The length is usually between three to five minutes, depending on the amount and quality of the material you have, but these numbers are not set in stone. It's better to have a short, concise one-and-a-half minute demo than a slow, leisurely five minutes. The selection and order of the scenes is based on the same value—quality. The scenes would be short, contain your best performances, with close-ups, and show you working with celebrities if possible. This is your tape and should reflect the best you possible, as an actor and a professional.

You'll choose a nice opening graphic with your name, maybe some brief intro music to begin, and then get right into the clips. A good editor will usually know the best order and way to highlight your work, but you're paying for the demo and shouldn't leave until you have the reel you want. The editor may then keep a copy of the work in a computer file for future reediting. That doesn't mean you are required to use that person again, but if you do, the original clips are already loaded and this could save you time and money. Through the years, you'll modify your reel to include newer and hopefully more substantial clips. And regardless of what happens with your demo, someday your grandkids will have a nice highlight reel of your career!

Dialects

Have you ever heard a Canadian actor try to do an American regional accent? It can rattle you. Have you ever heard an American try to sound like he's Cockney? To survive the world of dialects, you'd better have a great ear and some training, preferably both, or simply don't attempt to do one.

Dialects can be a great tool for the working actor, but they can also hinder you if you try to do one in front of a camera and you aren't able to pull it off. The best advice is that you should have a voice teacher who can help you to determine if you have the ability to deliver believable dialects. Then it's up to you to find out which ones you can do with aplomb. No actor can play every role and no actor can do all accents. You might be swell at southern twangs and even be able to find six different versions for that many regions south of the Mason-Dixon line, but that doesn't mean you'll be top notch doing a genuine New York borough accent.

If you can't do one, fine. Plenty of great actors have never tried to alter their voices to fit the regionalism of their characters. However, if you have the ability to add a vocal dimension to your role, it could be all the better for it. A voice teacher can take you a long way toward that goal, but you've got to have that gift of a good ear as your starting point. Most people that have this basic ability know it before they ever head to class to refine it. If you've already exhibited to yourself or your teacher the ability to get a genuine dialect going in time for shooting, then you might go for it. Otherwise, avoid it.

If you do move forward and it's not believable, the director will tactfully let you know. Speaking of which, if you have dialect down perfectly you can just do it, but if you're not sure you can query the director before you rehearse. He still may not want you to do it, but at least you've brought him into the decision. This shows respect.

Directors

If you're going to survive and succeed in Hollywood, you're going to have to learn to understand directors—their personalities, their needs, their vision, and their occasional quirkiness. Actors might get the rap for being colorful and eccentric, but I'd say directors give them a real run in this department.

Everything you've heard about film and television directors is true. The good ones are fun to work with, the bad ones can make your life misery, and the great ones remind you why you became an actor in the first place. There are geniuses and mediocre talents working within the industry.

Directors are brave and ambitious souls. Not only are they given the reins of a wild horse to control artistically, but they also are often technical masters. The technology constantly changes, and the best merge their hi-tech savvy with their creative juices to create wonderful things. There are actors' directors who are brilliant at coaxing great performances from thespians. And contrary to popular belief, they're not *always* the former actors. There are hardware directors who can make magic with the camera and with copious special effects but who aren't really attuned to actors. There are the ones who play both sides of the director's chair with equal aplomb. Then there are some who shouldn't be directing but they got the job anyway, so who are you to question?

How do you survive directors? There are plenty of ways, as unique as the person you're working for and the overall mood of the set. However, one common denominator applies for all occasions. Directors are incredibly busy, operating on many levels at the same time. They're setting up shots, catering to the star cast members, and troubleshooting with the cinematographer, producer, and head of every department. They're thinking about dialogue, wardrobe, and set pieces. They're wondering how much film they've shot and where the next set-up is and what time the Steadi-cam is being delivered. They have a lot on their plate and just a bit of time left over for the guest cast. So when they talk, you listen. You won't find too much attention being given to your element of the project. Sooner or later, the director will say something to you. It might just be, walk over there and say your line, but that's something. He likes you. He hired you and you're a professional, so walk over there and say your line. If you don't expect more, you'll fit in on a Hollywood set just fine. And sometimes, you'll get more attention than you think you deserve from a director. That's bonus time.

When it happens, listen even closer. He's giving you direction. If you pay attention, your performance will almost always be enhanced and the director will be your new friend for the day. Remember this person more than likely knows the entire story better than you do, so when he gives generously of his time to help guide you to better results you should take full advantage of it. You might even be encouraged to collaborate on something. The director might ask you, "What do you think this guy should be doing?" If that door is opened, step right in, but don't over extend your stay.

There are other kinds of sets where you might wonder whether the director even knows you're there in front of him. Once in awhile, you won't hear much other than the "Action" thing.

For survival's sake, do not let it bother you. It's usually just a result of the workload. Directors have to delegate. That delegating might mean you show up on set, are greeted by a wonderful assistant director who signs you in, sends you to make-up and wardrobe, delivers you to the set, introduces you to the cast members with whom you'll be acting, and then presents you to the director who nods and then walks past you.

Ouch. Don't take it personally. The director is busy getting the next shot, along with all those other details, before you'll fully appear on his radar. That usually occurs when it's your time to rehearse and when you will indeed get some attention. Some, being the key word. If it's a television show, this may be the first time the director has actually seen you in person so don't be too rattled if he regards you with no more than a blank stare. It's not that he doesn't like you. It's not that he doesn't respect actors. It's not that he's indifferent to your performance. If he's indifferent to your performance, then he'll let you know. Assuming he likes what you're doing, he may not say anything at all. Because no news is good news to a working actor, keep doing what you're doing if no one tries to stop you. You're doing your job well and giving the director one less headache for the day. That's a victory on some sets, so help the busy director out by knowing your lines, hitting your marks, and listening to everything he says even if you don't get a chance to do it just the way you did with your acting teacher the previous day. You're already way ahead of the game. You got the job, a nice paycheck, a trailer in which to stow your stuff, and a nice credit for your resume. Don't expect much more.

It's when you don't expect much more that you get just that. You'll show up to a very busy set, tons of activity happening simultaneously, multiple crisis's looming, everything's running well behind schedule, and just when you decide your best bet for survival is to steer clear of the bullets you'll get the grand treatment.

The director will pat you on the back, welcome you to the set, and ask you how you're feeling. What? Me? I'm not in this cast. I was brought in to say, "Here's your pizza, ma'am." Doesn't matter, you've found a great director who has left time for you, too. When he's done filming the regular who's playing the scene opposite you, he instructs the director of photography to line up a close-up of you. A close-up? For the pizza delivery guy? Have you hit the lottery? Yep. And he actually shoots the scene three times to give you a chance to play with your part a bit. That's a great day.

Then there are the days that aren't great. You're on a different set and the director hasn't even acknowledged your presence. He refers to you as the other actor when he's talking to the assistant director. When it comes time to shoot your coverage, he keeps the camera on you for about three seconds while scanning the room to keep up with his fluid camera style. After you've stood next to the camera to read your lines to the star on set who has done her work from six different angles about twenty times, he gives you one shot at your line reading before calling "moving on." Is that a bad day? No, not a great one either, but you were just acting on a professional set and that's a lot better than driving fifteen minutes to drop a headshot off to a casting director for the chance to work some day.

Then there are some rare but scathingly bad days. You're on set and doing exactly what you did in your audition. You notice that the director has been treating everyone rather badly and you've decided to stay out of his eye line until called to do your job. The chance never comes. In rehearsal, the director doesn't like what you're doing and he's not quiet about it. He wants to know why you're waving your hands when you say your lines. You tell him you won't do that anymore, he says you're right you won't, and before you know it you're heading outside the gate without a job. When you found out later the director was only throwing his weight around to impress the producer, you chalk it up to one of those bad days in Hollywood.

So you survive by listening, watching, and doing your job, appreciating that in the vast majority of cases the work is fast and when it's your turn you are expected to do it well and quickly. Anything else is icing on the cake. You read the mood of the set and the man who is running the set—the director. You might love him or hate him, agree or disagree with him, but he's your boss for as long as you're on that set and you'd better respect what he says. There's a lot written about television being a producer's medium and it is. The directors are jobbed in, different from episode to episode, and the producers are the ones who control the show week in and week out. Doesn't matter to you. The director is still the man for whom you must deliver. It might be the first sitcom the director has done, but he's Martin Scorcese to you and don't forget it. Because you're a smart actor, you also realize the producers have the power to make or break your day so everything I've said here about the director also applies to the producers.

You also survive by doing something that quite a few actors can't grasp. You don't make the director's job more difficult than it is already. You don't pester him, interrupt him, argue with him, or do anything that is less than gracious, professional, and expected.

For your professionalism, you'll be paid back in spades. You won't get cut, you'll have a nice clip for your reel, and you might even get the chance to work for that television director several times during your career.

Distractions

Los Angeles has more distractions than Idaho has potatoes. If you want to avoid focusing on your career, you can be sure to find all sorts of ways to make that happen. Look left, look right; there is plenty to help you keep your mind off acting. You like partying? We have nightclubs galore. You want to work on your tan or be a gym rat; you can pretty much do it year-round. You can spend complete days whiling away your time sitting in darkened theatres with wonderful stadium seating and perfect cup holders watching films from around the world. You can discover more trails to hike than you could ever hope to find. There are amazing museums that house international collections, dinosaurs, and even tiny miniatures. You can find casino gambling, strip clubs, new religions, and probably a class that's a combination of Tae Bo and Kabbalism if you want. There's cruising on the Pacific Coast Highway, shopping on Melrose, hanging at coffee bars on Sunset, and hitting Anaheim to overindulge yourself at numerous theme parks. You can sit in the desert and stare at the cactus all day, and then view the stars once the sun sets.

Some of these things you'll certainly want to do in your free time here in Los Angeles and you should, once you've taken care of business. Being our own bosses, it's easy to not take care of business first and that's when a career falters.

So the first question you should ask yourself each morning is, "Why have I come here?" Is it the museums, the view from Muholland, or the Mexican food? No, you came here to be a working actor. If you remind yourself of that when you're slacking off, it'll bring you back to the plan at hand. We all get distracted by LA's rainbow of options once in awhile, but surviving actors don't sail too far adrift for they know it'll only take them further away from their goals.

Down Cycles

Down cycles are one of the least written about realities of a surviving actor's career, and it's something I truly didn't comprehend until I'd lived here for awhile. My eyes were opened to the issue by an acting teacher who explained to me that there are periods of time when an actor gets cold for no apparent reason. I listened to the information, nodded, and didn't really apply it because I was in the midst of a tremendous year that I was sure would lead to an even better one the following year.

Guess what happened to me the following year? I couldn't get arrested. I wracked my brain for the reason. I was still studying, my acting was up to speed, I was getting enough auditions to warrant some work, and I was marketing myself as much as I had the last year. I couldn't for the life of me figure it out, but I kept pushing on.

Then I overheard two actors who reminded me of the wisdom my acting teacher had shared with me two years earlier. They were talking about the down cycles. My ears perked up. I started asking other actors about their cycles. I found out that almost every actor can be busy one year, perhaps flat or slow for a year or two, and then find they get hot again. What causes this actor phenomenon, and how do you survive it?

A common theory suggests that one gets over-auditioned in a certain period of time and falls off the casters' lists for awhile. Eventually the cycle ends when a casting director realizes she hasn't seen so and so in a long time and brings him into read. The actor gets a part and other casters see him working and think "maybe we should get him in here to read." Then the upswing cycle begins.

Maybe a down cycle occurred because a performer was overexposed. A popular commercial ran for a year and people got sick of seeing his face on TV every fifteen minutes. This happens, too. Everyone is familiar with television stars who are so overly associated with parts they've played that they do not work for years. This can happen to a lesser degree to unknown actors who might stand out for one job, particularly in the commercial world.

A down cycle can also arrive for no reason other than that your type fell out of fashion for a period. Or maybe you were working enough to not be overexposed but just enough to keep you from being aggressive in marketing for future work. There are numerous reasons it can happen, and professional actors know these things do end and then evolve into up cycles.

They seem to be inevitable and often are no fault of one's own. Down cycles aren't a reason to take two years off just because you figure it's your time to not get work and no one is going to hire you. You need to push on just as if it's your best year. You still study and work the instrument, market and keep the faith.

Then the up cycle comes back, you find yourself getting that first job in a long time, and the acting world is right again. Survive the down cycles and you'll endure a great part of the reason many actors quit. It's never easy, but when you begin to understand it's a universal fact of the business it becomes bearable.

E

Earthquakes

This is yet another subject in which you should take the term "survival" literally. Earthquakes are a fact of life for Californians. On occasion, the ground shakes and suddenly you realize you live on top of an ever-shifting Tectonic plate that has this peculiar inclination to move further North each year. Although they happen all the time, only rarely do you actually feel the earth move, and when you do feel it, it's one of those fun earthquakes.

By *fun* I mean the little common shaker that registers on the Cal State seismograph in the high 3s or low 4 range. Anything below that and you'd need to be a dog to even hear it. The ones you can actually feel happen a few times a year and are rarely awe inspiring. The first time you experience one you'll think a big truck just drove down your street and hit a pothole. Then you'll realize that was no truck but the earth shifting its weight. You'll grab the telephone to call your folks and tell them you are now an official resident of California.

Then there are those other kind of earthquakes. They are not fun. They're terrifying. I experienced one of the big ones during my very first week of residency in Los Angeles. No sooner had I arrived and found my very first apartment, when the Northridge earthquake of January 17, 1994, happened. This was the real deal—strong at 6.7, long, and life threatening. Believe me, it's an experience you don't want to have.

You'll probably never experience one that size, and tremblors (as some call them) will merely be the mild earth burping variety associated with the vast majority that occur. However, if you do happen to be here when a destructive quake hits, there are some survival tips that you'll need to know.

The old rule of thumb was that you should get under a sturdy door frame when a shaker occurs. However, they've pretty much changed their thinking on that one because so many people were getting hurt by swinging doors. The current thinking recommends getting under a solid desk or table, which will prevent things from falling on you. If you can't do that, at the very least move away from mirrors, glass, and other tall things that could fall on you. Another procedure some suggest is to head into the bathroom, although I don't understand the safety factor there, but a small room generally means structural soundness. If you're stuck in there for several hours, the convenience factor would certainly apply as well.

Electricity is sure to go out during big shakers but never light a candle to see your way around. Major quakes routinely break gas lines, and you know what happens when fire and gas meet. When you move here, purchase and keep flashlights in each room of your apartment or house. A battery-operated radio and fire extinguisher are musts. You'll find that home improvement and department stores sell various types of earthquake survival kits. They include first aid items, food stuffs, and other necessities. Buy a couple of those and put one in your bedroom and another somewhere else on your property. Like all smart Californians, keep an ample supply of bottled water at your place. If a worse-case scenario happens and you aren't able to get out for hours or even days, the water would be your lifeline.

There are all kinds of other earthquake tips on Internet sites. Pay at least one visit to these sites every year or so to get updated information that could save your life. The best one I've found is www.pasadena.wr.usgs.gov. Click on it and you'll find a lot of information you never knew about earthquakes, but first check out the preparedness area.

Preparedness is everything. Many earthquake experts also suggest you have a meeting place for you and your family members should you have to get out of your house. That makes sense, doesn't it?

Once you prepare for an earthquake, the first thing you should do is forget about them. The odds suggest you'll never face the danger of that worse-case scenario. You could even live here for years and never even feel that truck rumble by.

Energy

You need energy to be an everyday actor. You need it for a lot of reasons, not the least of which is that this is a very visual business. If you look low on energy, it'll hardly be an endorsement of your abilites. Working actors have great energy, and I'm not talking about the perpetually perky types, just professionals who are rested and focused in a good way, and ready for action. Walk into any audition room and you'll see a lot of this, but if you look around there'll be one or two people who look like they missed a good night's sleep. That can't be you.

Working out, getting plenty of rest, living a healthy lifestyle, partying in moderation only, and saving your energy for when you need it are all sensible approaches to your career in Los Angeles. A late night out before an audition will show. You might not think it will show, but it will.

Assuming you take care of yourself—body and mind—you'll project good energy when you walk into a roomful of producers. They like to hire people who have good, honest energy.

F

Feedback

Feedback is something that not every actor needs to hear. The fact of the matter is that a lot of good feedback doesn't lead to anything, and negative feedback can really mess with you if you don't learn to separate the significant comments from the stuff that is just a person's opinion.

If you do well at an audition, the casting director will probably tell your agent something generic like "she was good." That's nice to hear, but it isn't a substantial answer on the job you read for. It might not even help your agent get you back again. If you did fantastic, it might. If you don't do so well, your agent will probably hear nothing, unless she has a strong history with the casting director who will share this kind of sticky information.

The question is "do you really want to hear what people are saying about you?" Some actors do and others only take feedback when their agent broaches the subject. I keep mentioning your agent, because you will hardly ever get feedback directly from a casting director. They're just not going to do that, and you shouldn't expect it.

With your agent acting as the middle man, you might receive some valid feedback that can help you the next time out. Even if it's something negative, you can learn from it and do better the next time. It's a very subjective thing, too, so your agent won't toss you from the client list for one or two feedback bits that don't make you sound like a great actor. Just try to keep those numbers very low. A good agent will take the feedback and make a mental note of it. If they see a pattern forming, you will find out soon enough.

If you do solicit information, then be prepared to hear some stuff you're not going to like. There is no way you are going to impress everyone. You could go to one casting director and they'll love you and march you right over to producers. Another may be completely unimpressed with your acting. If you insist on hearing all reports that your agent gets, you will eventually find one that doesn't suit you. That's why I ask you to consider whether you need to even hear the feedback.

Agent Patty Grana-Miller offers this on the subject: "Sometimes you can get some very valid feedback. Always take it with a grain of salt. There are some things you can change, and some things you can't, and some things that are just about a difference in taste."

Film Auditions

Film auditions aren't dramatically different from those you'll experience for television shows, but there are a few things that do stand out about them. Most significant is that you often get more prep time than you'd experience in fast-paced TV land. It's common to have several days to a week to get ready after a casting director calls to set up a film reading time slot.

A smart actor won't let this opportunity go to waste. You'll use this bonus time to study the material, develop the character, and come up with a killer audition. It also affords you ample hours to work with an acting coach if you so choose. On many projects, the entire script is available for perusal; this is something many actors don't take the time to seek out. It's one thing if you're reading for a one- or two-line part, but if your role is any larger you can only be in a better position by having read the full text of the script.

You'll almost always pre-read for film parts and occasionally be put on tape. More often than not it'll just be you and the casting director at the first call and perhaps an assistant will be reading opposite you. If you do the right thing and are reasonably close to the type they are seeking, you may be invited back for a callback at a later date, where you'll almost always meet the director face to face and read for him. Unlike in television where the callbacks are often in front of many people, film, although normally of much larger budgets, is more intimate in the audition phase.

Fewer actors are present at film auditions than you'd find at television shows. Don't worry, they see plenty of talent for every role available, but the scheduling allows for less crowded waiting rooms. You may be the only actor there or they'll be a few others, but either way it's as relaxing an atmosphere as you could expect for an audition.

Because film has a longer casting process, you might not know for weeks if you are going to be brought back to meet with the director. Actors accustomed to television and commercial work are used to knowing within a few days, maybe the same day, if they are a contender for the part. Not here, so you'd be wise to learn to let auditions fade from your conscious once you're done. The alternative is that you'll be thinking about it over and over again. Actors tend to drive through red lights when they get this way. That's not good.

Another thing you'll find more often in film reads than television is the chance to read for multiple characters. Especially in films with many roles, it is not uncommon for a casting director to ask you to audition for two or more parts. The chances are higher for this happening in direct correlation to the size of the part. But it works in reverse. The smaller the part, the better chance you'll read for other roles, too. If you're trying to get a major role, they'll usually only have you come in for that one part.

If you receive a callback and meet the director and maybe a producer or two, you'll sometimes find a nice long audition. The director will often work with you, give you adjustments, and may have you read the part multiple times. In television, it's once maybe twice at the most. You should also know that anytime in any audition for any medium, when a director asks you to do it again, he really likes what you're doing.

This is just a quirky thing I've noticed through the years, but often you are told that you don't need to bring your headshot to a film audition. However, you should always bring it in case they don't have one on file. In commercials and quite often in television, they are missing your headshot. It happens here too. Better to be safe than sorry.

Freelancing

Although you'll read in some publications that freelancing is nonexistent in Los Angeles, there are indeed hundreds and hundreds of cases of actors working with agencies yet not signed under a formal contract. It happens all the time. Whether it be because the agent wants to try out the new talent to see what the market will bear or because the signed client list is already overburdened, there are many instances of this practice. However, this is very different than freelancing as it is done in New York City, where you work with multiple agencies at the same time. That wouldn't fly in Los Angeles.

Here you can certainly freelance, but it's an *exclusive* freelancing situation. In other words, the agent won't give you the one-year contract but she will submit you for roles. She won't call to clear you either as in New York and, in fact, if you try to work with another agent for the same jurisdiction, the first agent will drop you like a hot potato. You are only freelancing in that you aren't signed to a contract. Otherwise, you're treated pretty much like any other client of the agency. Have no fear. Once you start booking work, they'll put a contract in front of you faster than a mouse in a roomful of cats.

G

Getting Cut

Face it right now, you will get cut. If you are a professional actor working in film or television, it's only a matter of time before your favorite scene starring you will be chopped out of the final project. It might be because of time constraints (very common), story problems (semicommon), technical glitches, or performance issues (not too common), but it happens to every actor some time in his career.

A surviving actor will learn quickly never to take it personally when his scene is eliminated from the final edit. Talk to any working actor, all the way up to star level, and he'll have at least one or two cut stories. Usually it's pieces of a scene(s) that get cut and other times it'll be a whole scene or maybe even a whole character.

Sometimes it's better to play it safe and not to announce television appearances to friends and family until after the fact. The most depressing thing is announcing an appearance and then having the scene go AWOL. This doesn't mean you don't promote an appearance on the screen. You do, to casting directors. If the scene makes the edit, great, if not the CD will surely understand that the scene was nipped, and they won't hold it against you as they know cuts happen every hour of every day from good actors for things they've cast. Contrary to popular belief, it's not always just bad scenes that get cut. In fact, sometimes the best scenes get cut. The acting may be fantastic, the lighting and sound superb, and yet it just doesn't work in the context of the whole show, so out it goes.

A good friend of mine who is a busy working actor was invited to attend the big premiere of a feature film in which he'd played a nice role. He was given several passes and took his mother and wife. The red carpet, the search lights, the whole Hollywood premiere glitz. It was going to be a special event and the director, who had become a pal to the actor during filming, made sure to include him on the guest list.

Only one problem, my friend had been cut from the finished film. He found out as he sat there in the audience waiting for his scene to appear. It didn't. The director apologized for the mix-up and later explained that some time-constraint cuts were needed at the last minute so my buddy's role had been dropped from the film. Was my pal devastated? No, as a professional performer he's all too aware that these things happen. Sure his ego was bruised, as happens to us all sometimes, but that's showbiz and he rolled with it. It wasn't all bad. His name still ended up in the credits, which meant he'd see residuals for years to come. Even better, the director hired him in his next film (in a scene that made it to the big screen) and will undoubtedly use this talented guy again throughout the years.

Having your scene cut happens. Although you can't take it personally, it's not a pleasant experience, as I found out a few years back. I had more than a sneaky suspicion this one was coming because it was truly only one of two times I've worked with a director I didn't like. Before the episode aired, I figured I better confirm my suspicions. I called the production company to inquire how I might get a copy of the scene. The very friendly editor's words were, "You know, we really loved that scene." I knew from the past tense of the word *love* that my scene wasn't going to be on the network a few nights later. The credit still remained on my resume for a few months. Hey, I'm not stupid.

Giving Back

There's something I believe as important to an actor's success as a good headshot and resume—giving back. As tough as the acting business is, we are truly privileged to be able to do it. For whatever reason you are here, you must know that some kind of karmic divine intervention played itself out in your life that gave you the opportunity to pursue a career as an actor. Even when we're in our worst periods as actors, we are still so blessed to see the uniqueness and almost unexplainable beauty in the simple act of being a performer—even an unemployed one. We are lucky to be here doing this!

So why not pay that back.

There are tons of ways to give back. Some actors dedicate themselves to improving the lives of their fellow thespians. In recent years, in particular, some very high-profile successes have literally put their careers on hold so that they can run for office in SAG. Others speak publicly to government officials or any media outlet about the plight of performing in twenty first-century America. Everyone can do something.

Two years ago during the commercial strike, I was marching down Wilshire Boulevard with several thousand actors, most whose names you wouldn't recognize, but there among them were the big names, too.

David Hyde Pierce happened to be marching right next to me and using his celebrity to further the cause. Did he need to be there? No, he's made a major name for himself. He's done films and, of course, became the Niles we all know and love on "Frasier." He certainly could have stayed away from this march, but he gave back.

You don't have to be a celebrity to help out with charities, but if you do hit it big, find a cause and throw some weight around for the right reasons. Do something big with that A-list name of yours to draw attention to the cause. Love it or hate it, we live in a world that listens to people who are successful at acting, signing, and tossing a basketball. If you get that kind of success, give it right back with your good deeds.

Sometimes it's just bad karma to not give back. You could share some time and experience with a newer actor or someone looking for guidance. That's just as important. I know one actor who struggled for years. A lot of people helped him. Then he achieved great success in a particular area. He's very busy now. Not long ago, I asked him to answer a question or two to an aspiring young actor. You know what his answer was? "Tell her to stay away. There's no work." It wasn't followed by a chuckle and real information. That's called not giving back.

Whatever you do, marching in a union parade, instructing a new actor on some pitfalls to avoid, volunteering to read with another actor in preparation for a role, running for office, or just being a gracious actor to your fellow thespians, you must give back. It's your duty. Ignore that duty as some do and you most certainly will be missing out on a grand opportunity for betterment. Selfishness might not keep you from success, but at what cost have you achieved it? Acting is important but not as important as your humanity.

Going Up On Lines

Everybody forgets their lines once in awhile. It's okay, and you'll survive it. As long as you know what to do in the different places in which it might happen—pre-reads or first auditions, callbacks, or during actual performance on set.

Let's discuss auditions first. Sometimes lines go right out the window, so if you mess up your dialogue, here's what to do. Stop and ask if you can start again. That's not rocket science. That's okay for auditions when you are reading perhaps a few lines to maybe ten. If you're doing a long scene and you get through two minutes of it before you mess up, then it's probably not fortuitous to stop and ask to go again. Let it ride and push on, just like you would if you were in a live performance on stage. If you go completely blank, you still have your script sides to fall back on.

Casting directors are very supportive people, especially when they have the time to be so in a pre-read situation. As long as you are polite, they'll almost always give you a second chance to do it—possibly even a third if they believe you're right for the role. This doesn't mean you dare go in there unprepared. You're a professional actor and they expect you to do your homework. The actors before and after you probably did, and so should you.

Forgetting lines because of nerves is a different thing. Prepared or not, it can still happen. It can be most unsettling if you mess up lines at a callback in front of the whole creative team. At this second audition, you would definitely ask to start again only if it happened at the very beginning. Callbacks are always run on fairly tight schedules. There are a lot of actors brought in in quick succession and there is just no time to repeat performances. Do your best. If you get into the body of the piece and drop lines, don't look to them with "deer in the headlight" eyes. Take a breath, look down at your script, and get right back into it. Sometimes a recovery can be as impressive as a good reading. You're not the first actor to forget a line in a pressure situation.

On set you are in full performance mode. Once in awhile you will forget a line. In television they are often rewriting things right up until the end, so you may barely have a chance to memorize the lines you'll forget! Be a pro. Working actors learn to adapt and apply changes quickly. If you mess up a line, don't stop, laugh, or yell cut. The director yells cut. The stars can laugh when they mess up, not you. Push on and don't count on getting another chance to do it in Take two. You may mess up the line and end up with something that works just as well. The director and producer may not even care. If you stray too far from the words, the writer will care, so do your best.

If the director does stop the scene because you are so off course as to make it unworkable, a short sorry is all you need to offer. Then you do it again and better the next time. Most times though, if you transpose a word or forget one line of many, it won't make much of a difference. You keep acting until someone tells you to stop. If the line(s) you drop are integral, the script supervisor will make sure you know to put them in the next take. The bottom line is, if you're doing good acting work, they will forgive an occasional line mess up. *Occasional* is the operative word here.

Good Stuff

You put up with a lot of difficult stuff if you stick it out as an actor. Most auditions don't result in work, most days don't even offer up a tangible sign of a forward-moving career, and you're always in a field that offers no promises.

But then there is good stuff, and I'm here to tell you if you work hard, make good contacts, and are ready when the opportunity comes, you will get your shots at working. You can take that work as far as it will allow you to go; the sky is the limit. There are wonderful days as an actor and they come when you least expect them.

Maybe it's been a slow three months; you've had a grand total of one audition and it was for a laxative. Hardly the "Streetcar Named Desire" you played the lead in in college. Then your pager goes off. It's not even your agent, probably one of those workshops calling to try and get you to buy their class right? Wrong, it's a casting director, and he's calling you directly. You didn't even think the guy knew your name let alone your phone number, but he knows both—that's part of his job. He wants you to come in the next morning for a producer call for a popular sitcom. He's not even requiring a pre-read. It turns out that his assistant called you in a few years ago for an audition for another show and still had your picture in his files in a whole new office.

You readily accept the audition and tell him your new agent's name. He tells you he'll fax the sides right away to you. What, you don't even have to pay to get them? Nope. He's taking care of it right now. You get your audition time, thank him, and begin calling your agent even before he's off the line.

Your agent is actually pleased to hear from you, undoubtedly because you're bringing good news. You explain how the caster called you directly and you just wanted to let her know what happened. She thanks you for taking care of the arrangements and compliments you on making the audition happen. Make it happen? You were watching a rerun of "All In The Family" for the thirtieth time.

The sides are now coming across your fax machine and the role is actually meaty. Maybe it's not a major guest star who is dating the show's lead but it's a nice part—a nice part dropped from heaven into your lap, if you can deliver at the audition.

The next day you arrive at the audition site and find only four other actors waiting to read. That's all they've brought in for the part. After a slow period and one that had followed a series of major league cattle calls, you are happy to see you have a decent chance for a part. The other actors smile warmly as you walk in and there is none of that weird audition waiting room stuff you've encountered from time to time. As you sit and wait for the producers to arrive, the casting director comes out and offers everyone a water or coffee and thanks you for patiently waiting for the team to show.

Patient? Thank me? We've only been here for five minutes. Thank you for thinking of us out of a gazillion performers who would welcome any audition call. Thank you very much.

The caster tells the room that he really appreciates everyone coming in on such short notice and that they'll be making a decision right after the audition. They'd like everyone to hang around and then they'll book someone after all five have read.

Then he walks back into the office and you have nice conversation with the other actors—and you don't even talk about all the shows for which you've read. You talk about the weather, the Lakers or about the little puppy who rescued its owner from a runaway weed wacker—anything but acting. You like this group of performers so much that you release the full want of the role. Okay, you need the job so maybe you hold onto just a bit of it, but you're feeling is that anyone who gets it deserves it. And that feeling is coming right back to you. One guy even cracks, "Hey, there's twenty lines right? Why don't we take four each and share the gig?" Everyone laughs, wishing we had that option.

The producers come in, say hello to everyone, and then disappear into the same room as the caster.

You're called in first. Ooooh, that's a toughie. Most actors prefer going late in the audition, but an audition is an audition and who cares when you go? The executive producer jumps out of his sofa seat and shakes your hand. You should be jumping up to shake his hand but you're already standing. He, too, thanks you for coming in on such short notice. Are you kidding? You would have stolen a car to get here.

Then they tell you to go ahead whenever you want. You do the bit and get some big laughs at the right moments. It's all going exceedingly well, so you decide to make a broad choice for the last line—something that was in your best-case scenario audition thought process. There is a long pause after you said it as if they're taking it all in and one huge burst of laughter—it worked. They thank you and ask you to wait outside while they read the rest of the guys.

You walk back out and one actor says, "Sounds like you got 'em good?"

"No," you say, "just warming them up for you." And you were. You sit down and he goes in and the laughter from inside is deafening. He's killing them. He walk out laughing and sits down and gives a "who knows" look. He tells the next actor—nice people in there. He's right.

The scene is repeated another three times. Each actor that goes in gets big laughter and comes out looking like a million bucks. If we could only all get the role together, it would be a great set. When the last actor comes out, someone says "Hey, whoever gets the gig, good job." Then the conversation is back to talking about the knitting club that hit the lottery last week—interesting metaphor.

Who gets the role? It doesn't matter. It wasn't about the result. It's about the experience of a good day. A day you got to do what you do; be a professional actor. The job would be nice, too, but the audition, the camaraderie, and the professionalism is what you have to appreciate. The result is a bonus. I was there and it was a great day to be an actor.

H

Headshots

The headshot is your first and continual method of introducing and reintroducing yourself to agents, casting directors, and other powers in the entertainment field. A good part of your survival is going to be in the type and quality of headshot you use to market with. It's not a science and it's often very subjective, but a good headshot—even if people don't always agree on what about it makes it work—will take you a long way. Remember though, once you're called in to audition because of that picture, you have to deliver the goods. That's why it's important for newer actors not to rush out and spend money for a headshot session until their acting and auditioning skills are up to a professional level.

Headshot styles seem to change about every five or six years—from close-ups, to three-quarter body shots, and then back again. Whatever stylistic preference comes in and out of vogue, there are really only two things that surviving actors must concern themselves with in regard to their 8×10.

First, the picture must look like you. That seems pretty obvious, yet so many actors make the mistake of showing someone else in their pictures. Hollywood already has somebody else, give them you. If you try to airbrush yourself to glamour queen beauty or make yourself look thinner than you are, you are in for a lot of aggravation. If you're fifty, you shouldn't try to appear as if you're thirty. Average-looking people shouldn't try to doctor up their headshots into movie star handsome. Just be yourself and have your picture reflect that.

Every casting director will tell you the same thing. The picture must appear as you appear in real life. They wouldn't need to repeat this if there weren't a lot of people ignoring the obvious. When you walk in the door to meet a caster, producer, or talent representative, you don't want them to look at you, at the picture, and then back at you and have an "is this you" look on their face. That's not a good look.

Be smart by not misrepresenting yourself. Listen to commercial casters Robert and Jacob Ferret wax philosophic on the subject.

Jacob: It's like a short, chubby guy trying to make himself a Brad Pitt type in his headshot. It's not going to happen, whether he believes it or not.

Robert: More women do it than men. We'll be casting for a 32-year-old woman, who looks natural and real.

Jacob: And they're headshot looks like they're 32.

Robert: Then they come in to audition and they're 45. And you're like, what the hell? How *old* is this picture? They're completely different. We'll call the agent and go, "Have you seen this person lately?"

Survival means using some common sense because most people aren't going to invest themselves in you enough to tell you that your headshot looks like a completely different person. They're going to smile, let you read, and then probably never bring you in again. Actors that have been doing this for awhile need to remember that their picture must look like them today, not ten years ago when they guest starred on "TJ Hooker." Some veterans make the mistake of holding onto a headshot that has worked for them for many years. It might be a great one, but if its day has passed it's time for a new sitting.

Second, the picture must be of professional level and in focus. It seems silly to have to write that, but amateurish headshots are all over the place. Soft images, pictures shot by the actor's friend in the backyard, and all kinds of other bad images are around. What does that say about how you regard your image and your career?

Spend the money to get professional shots from a headshot photographer who makes his living in the business, get your lithographs run off at the best printer, and send them out.

Most actors work with at least two or three different headshots at any given time. The standard rule of thumb is a minimum of two. There is the theatrical shot, which shows the actor in some manner of serious look and thought. It could be thoughtful, pensive, smoldering, or scary, but not giddily happy. Actors tend to have a couple theatrical shots to use for different projects. You probably wouldn't submit a shot of you in sport coat for a role as a construction worker, but you would use that when submitting for the part of a detective. Whatever number of theatrical shots you use in Los Angeles, the picture should reflect the types of characters you would normally play. Sometimes you have to take the guess work out of the equation to get them to bring you in.

The other predominant picture is the commercial headshot, which is very clean-cut, preppy, and advertiser friendly, featuring you with a nice smile and no hint of anything going on but pure happiness. In commercials, you're supposed to convince people to buy things. A friendly young dad, caring mom, or warm face of the always quirky next door neighbor is what the advertising world usually goes for, and most pictures lean that way. Of course, in these days of anything goes in the commercial world, you will find a wide variety of charactery, bizarre, and nonsmiling shots popping up on casting desks all over town. So if you look like an intimidating prison inmate, there's probably no reason for you to try to smile like a toothpaste model. You won't be getting called in for those parts anyway.

From an agent's standpoint, the picture has to be able to sell you as much as the talent representative who is messengering it all over town. Kurt Patino, a film and television agent at the Bobby Ball Agency in Los Angeles, knows first hand about the significance of finding the right shot:

> Your headshot is your most important tool to get you in the door. Capturing the perfect headshot is like painting the perfect picture. Metaphorically speaking, you might have to keep painting the landscape until you have something that shines and holds someone's attention. If it's not working, shoot again . . . and again . . . and again, until you have something that gets you into the room. Always have enough money saved to get new shots. Keep refining your look until it turns into something marketable.

Although your headshot must be of that great quality, you needn't go overboard in reproducing it. Lithographs are very inexpensive and are the accepted method for mass reproduction of headshots and postcards. Most actors get three to five hundred lithos done at a time for a very reasonable price (well under $100 at most printers). A litho made from the original can be copied with minimal loss to the picture quality. A few actors make the mistake of ordering photo originals, which are exorbitantly priced (over $1 a piece). Don't throw your money away. If the work has been shot digitally, each picture printed will be an original and there will be no loss in picture quality whatsoever.

Hitting a Mark

Although they should, they don't teach you about hitting marks in college acting classes. You generally find out about their importance when you arrive on a set and find that an intricate camera move in a pivotal scene in the film relies almost exclusively on making sure you hit the spot on the ground that has been predetermined to be your mark.

The camera that films you has a lens, and the only image that'll end up in the picture is what fits in it. You might have a safer zone when they're using a wide angle, but when they tighten up you'd better be exactly where you're supposed to be on repeated takes.

You've got other things to think about: your lines, your acting, speaking clearly, maybe working with a major star who doesn't like to do more than one or two takes, or a producer who is looking at his watch because he's already fifteen minutes into meal penalties. Then you search the floor and see a tiny piece of tape that you'd better end up on after you walk the distance of a room during your scene. That's your mark. Hit it, pal. No pressure there, huh?

Everybody misses their mark from time to time; if you keep a sense of humor, you'll survive it when it happens to you. The most pragmatic piece of advice I can offer comes from a very consistent method of hitting a mark—the reverse step count. When they put your mark on the ground, if they can for camera, it'll be a beautiful little t-shaped piece of tape. If you're standing still during the scene you have no problem. Step on the tape and do your stuff. It gets trickier if you have to walk into the spot. Here's what you do. Walk backward from the spot to where your start mark is off camera. Count the steps. Then do it again, and maybe a third time if you can. Take normal size steps and don't get overly conscious of how far apart your steps are. Your body will come through for you if you let it. If all goes well you'll hit the mark each time when you walk forward an equal number of steps. Now you can also cheat a bit. If it's a fairly tight shot and the camera is favoring the other actor when you walk to your mark you can subtly, very subtly, glance down. Don't do this if the camera is on your face.

Sometimes they can't put a piece of tape on the ground because it'll show up on film. In that case, you have a couple of different options. If you're shooting outside, you can use any natural item, such as a twig or a rock. If you're indoors and there is nothing that could discriminately be used, you can employ another method of mark hitting altogether. I'll call it centering.

During rehearsal when you establish where you are to end up, find a visual on which you can center. Let's say you're on a hospital set. Standing there at your final mark, what do you see? Don't count on the other actor because he might miss his mark. Is there a poster hanging in front of you, or maybe a lamp on a table a few inches from your hand? There are hundred of things you can find to help guide you to your mark. It's best to locate something that's at eye level in the direction you are going to be looking. It's there. Center yourself on the item or on part of the item—whatever works best for your position. Re-create that position each time. It works.

Hype

One night after a long day of writing this book, I came home, plopped down in my favorite chair, and clicked the TV remote. As I was scanning the way we men do (forty channels in forty seconds), I stopped on a show that I've never seen an entire episode of, "Entertainment

Tonight." I watched almost in horror at the stories they had on there. It was LA night and there was an exposé on plastic surgery gone awry, a day in the life piece following some former bodybuilder hottie who is trying to make herself into a movie star, and yet another exploitative segment that chronicled some Hollywood celeb as she got ready for a court appearance. Highbrow stuff obviously! I realized that nearly each segment in its own way was designed as yet another glamour/scandal exposé, and I also thought this has nothing at all to do with life in the real Los Angeles. It was pure hype.

That stuff is out there I guess, but when you're here being a professional actor, that sort of "other-plane Hollywood" is something you just don't see. It's a creation like the movies that are made here. People all over the United States still hold onto the perception of LA as a pretty wacky place, and it has its moments, but basically it's a fairly blue-collar, go to work, and come home kind of town. The bright lights and special effects are a real part of the workday for a percentage of the population, but that's not who they are or how they live. LA is just another city—a very pretty city with a lot to see and do—not that other place they show you on ET and in *People* magazine. That's created for the cameras. I'm not saying there aren't a few stereotypes mixed in, but you only see them enough to remind you that they actually exist. You could probably seek out and find more of that stuff if you really searched it out, but that seems like a real waste of time.

You're here to be an actor and a real person so don't buy into the hype. Hype exists only to sell tickets. If you hit your wildest dreams and have all the success you can take, that's a great thing. Like so many other major celebrities, you probably don't have to have a camera crew following you to the bathroom, nor a phalanx of bodyguards to escort you 24/7. Keep it real. Most professionals do.

I

Inexperience

I hope if you're reading this book as a new arrival to Los Angeles that you've come here with some genuine acting experience. I don't mean a play in high school or the ability to do a great DeNiro impression at the company picnic. I'm talking professional experience. That's training, auditions, credits, and having existed as a making-your-living-at-it actor somewhere else.

This is no place for a beginner. Survival in LA is tough for actors with experience, credits, and contacts. It's nearly impossible for someone who doesn't possess those things. Yet because this is the mecca of entertainment, there are plenty of hopefuls who ignore common sense and plunge in headfirst putting their dream ahead of common sense.

Hollywood has a reputation for hiring looks over talent, and they do indeed like to book the beautiful and young, but what you don't know are that those precocious kids and perfect model-turned-actresses who turn up so frequently on television are often veterans of other acting markets. They came here seasoned and ready to compete. If those who fall in the ideal casting demographic needed experience first, then you'd better bring it too if you expect to have any shot here.

Yet it's a common mistake so many newcomers make—rushing here too soon. No skills, no resume, and no knowledge of the business. Then adding insult to injury they immediately try to find acting work when they should be looking for an acting class. That's a very bad plan. Blame Hollywood for it if you must—for the "anybody can be discovered here syndrome" lives on in media hype. Yes, people are discovered all right. They're called professional actors, and they previously appeared in regional theatre in Sarasota, television commercials in Seattle, and industrial films in Minneapolis before they tried this place. Common sense would suggest anyone would follow that kind of lead.

The letters always arrive at the "Tombudsman" desk from inexperienced actors craving the acting life, as if wishing for it were enough to make it happen. Those who have been here for three weeks are usually wondering where to get a good headshot and an agent so they can start work. Those who have been around three months are perplexed because they can't seem to get an appointment with anyone in town. The letters from those who have been sitting around for a year or two without a clue as to what to do are usually from inexperienced people that came here without a foundation to build upon.

If you're here already but lacking the skills essential to the environment, you'll have to work that much harder. Casting director Jeff Gerrard has this to offer:

> You must train, learn, listen and network, and do not go out on auditions until you are ready. Many years ago when I was an actor someone told me "You'll get in the doors, but you want those doors to stay open for you." So what you want to do is make sure you are ready to be in there.

Why is it that so many have trouble putting that training concept first? It's because Hollywood has never been about promoting the unglamorous elements of acting. No one is doing an exposé on acting classes and the thousands of people who attend them weekly. It's much more fun to highlight a story about someone fresh off the bus who got into a television series. Remember hype? Working doctors train. Working accountants train. So do plumbers, lawyers, athletes, carpenters, cinematographers, and directors. Why would actors be any different?

Acting teacher Daphne Eckler Kirby sees the same thing and has a cogent theory as to why people continue to jump in before they should:

> Because acting is an art form that when done well looks very easy, and all of us who do it know it's a very difficult craft, some actors are jumping into the business end before their work is ready. And if they're lucky enough, which can happen if they have a special look, they go out and audition and the work is not of the quality to get them even in the ballpark of being booked or called back. What can happen then is a downward spiral because the casting director will tell the agent that the actor is green and the agent might lose interest in the actor based on that.

So learn elsewhere. Baltimore, Atlanta, Miami, Chicago, Seattle, Boston, Dallas, Philadelphia—every region has a city where there are ample professional opportunities to train and learn. Use them. Build a resume elsewhere and get on-stage, and hopefully even some on-set, experience before you come to Los Angeles. Exhaust those opportunities before even thinking of this place. You'll be a much better positioned actor for it and vastly increase your chances for a future in this sunny but very tough city.

Internet-itis

The Internet has finally taken over the world officially since both your Grandmother and four-year-old sister are surfing the Internet in different rooms at the same time. It's also made its presence felt in our acting industry, and there are some places it really can help a career and others where the theory is better than the reality.

That's why I call this section Internet-itis. There are lots of Web sites but only some are worthy of your attention. A sixteen-year-old kid with a good computer can make a Web site that'll rival Yahoo, but that doesn't mean the information on it will help your acting career. The Internet has hundreds of Web sites about acting and your challenge is in separating the helpful from the frivolous.

For research about the acting field, the Internet is, at times, fantastic. There are so many Web sites that inform, protect, and serve actors that the forever promise of "ten years from now" is already here. These Web sites are particularly good for their message boards and chat areas, which offer everything from career advice, audition listings, and even to suggesting which industry people to meet and which to avoid. Just by offering a community for actors—neophyte through veteran—and taking the isolation out of the profession the Internet has empowered many performers in many ways.

Everyone is sharing information, and aside from the occasional silliness that comes from a world where comments and articles can be posted fairly anonymously, much of what makes it to your screen is surprisingly accurate, informative, and occasionally eye opening. Although actors will always be competing with each other for work, the Internet has also fostered a sense of camaraderie in a traditionally solitary field. There's a movement of "I'll help you with what I know, you help me with what you know, and everyone benefits."

Many of these Web sites are run by very knowledgeable performers and quality organizations—others by people who are just too far out there to follow. Smart surfing will help you figure out which sites are legit and which make a strong argument for free Web space being given to anyone with dial-up access.

So the Internet is already booming on the acting research front. However, the early excitement about the web centered on the concept of bringing together actors, agents, and casting directors in some vision of a utopian interconnection. You almost expected to see one of the monkeys from "2001 A Space Odyssey" tossing his own headshot into space.

It's hardly that in 2002. Although big money from some highly publicized entities has been pumped in and often lost since the 1990s, the Internet has never become the great answer for actors in regard to promoting their faces. Performers still predominantly do their submissions through postal mailings and dropoffs of 8×10s and postcards. Casting directors still cast by opening up those countless manila envelopes. Agents still submit their clients through messengered photo deliveries and the occasional fax, and by working the phones. Maybe in the *next* ten years, it'll finally become the vision so many predicted earlier, but today marketing, casting, and agenting are still done, with a few isolated exceptions, the good old-fashioned way.

Another side of the actor Web is performers posting their headshots and video clips for anyone and everyone to peruse. That's nice, but how many people in the hiring world have time to look or are inclined to look at these things? Not many for now, although some casters admit to going to the Web when they've exhausted their search for some specialty actor—like a unicyclist who can recite Shakespeare. For the rest of us, we'll see what the future brings.

So use the Internet to network a bit, pick up a few tips, and learn about what's going on in the industry but don't dump your money into startup ventures that promise you exposure to the powers that be. Get some more headshots done, take another acting class, and give your agent a call to see *what* they're submitting you for. You won't have to worry about the how.

Is It Really Worth It?

I wouldn't have written this book if I didn't think it was.

Sure acting is hard, even harder in Los Angeles, and yes, it's an unfair business. There's absolutely no doubt that talent is sometimes pushed aside in favor of appearance. There are things about acting that will always have you scratching your head.

Then comes your turn to show what you've got. You get your teeth into a good role, find a film set that is full of energy and talent, or join a company of like-minded actors in a new theatre company that breathes new life into your soul. And it gets better each time.

Acting is so worth it.

The key is surviving the stuff that makes you wonder in the first place. If we could act all the time, the question would likely never arise, but we can't. We are in a profession of part-time performance, sometimes part part-time. Instead, we pursue full time and during that pursuit we come up against a slew of things that force us to question what we do—unemployment and charlatans being the big two.

But those things aren't acting. They are just items we have to work around to get to the good stuff. So when you get frustrated, for whatever reason, bring it back to the work. That's why you're doing this after all. Laugh the other stuff off and think about the last time you played the part. Remember the light on your face, the actor you worked with, and the incredible feeling of "present momentness" that swept over you. I know you've felt that. We all do. You put something good out there, something that was pure and unselfish. That's why you do it, and you'll continue to do it. The next time is only just around the corner.

J

Jaded

You'll need to avoid becoming jaded if you are going to survive and succeed in Hollywood. There are so many ways to become jaded in this city and industry, and it's something that happens to enough people that it deserves attention here.

It most often rears its ugly head because of the competition factor. Some make great progress in their career and some don't, and some of those who don't get frustrated. Frustration repeated over time can easily lead to a jaded attitude.

Hollywood does not always reward stick-to-it-ness and in that shuffle of new product day in and day out people with experience and credits sometimes get pushed aside for someone younger, better looking or better connected. You cannot change that aspect of the business, but you can avoid becoming jaded about it if you choose. Every working actor and star in Hollywood knows how this town likes to use up the product and put something new on the shelf. That's a tough reality of this television and film field. Today's television star is often later unemployed and back to auditioning in a few years. Many actors don't make it that far, and they witness other people achieving positive things all the time.

Don't over think it. It has nothing to do with your career. Your neighbor down the hall landing a series will not keep you from a great future. The untalented guy from acting class who miraculously lands a big role in film won't make it harder for you to do the same. Some common complaints of the jaded or near jaded are, "Oh, I'm not playing that game," or "It's got nothing to do with talent, it's who you know." It's nonsense. Jadedness, for whatever reason, is only an excuse for not doing better.

Joining SAG

The Screen Actors Guild is a major influence and power in the film and television industry. For all its faults and infighting of recent years, it remains a dominant force. You, as an actor, want to be inside that power, and as these things work out, you will be eventually.

Don't, however, make it the sole focus of your early career, because becoming a member is hardly a guarantee of success. Nationally, there are over 98,000 current members of SAG. Sixty percent identify themselves as residing in the Los Angeles area. Very few of these people are steadily working actors. Most have second or third jobs to support their acting career, and you'd be amazed at the amount of professionals who would be happy just having enough gigs to qualify for health insurance. There will always be many more prospective employees than there are jobs to be had even in this center of entertainment, but you don't want to rush into SAG until you are genuinely good and ready.

Yet, so many actors new to Los Angeles often make getting into SAG their number one priority. Some pros are eligible to join because they've done principal work under an AFTRA contract. A year after a speaking role under AFTRA and SAG will welcome you to the fold. Others get in after collecting a few vouchers through doing extra work. This process can take a week or years, depending on the luck and or persistence of the nonunion extra. On more than a few occasions, a producer will simply insist on a nonunion actor for a part in his SAG project. That actor gets right in. A few sneak into SAG through illegal means; the most common way is by paying a fee to someone to get them the three vouchers to join SAG. For an organization that has a reputation among outsiders as being terribly difficult to join, plenty seem to be joining. In fact, SAG keeps taking them in despite the fact that employment will only be had by relatively few of the members. SAG makes big bucks through its membership regardless of whether you ever work. As soon as a new recruit finds a way, he'll rush over to the SAG office on Wilshire Boulevard, plop down close to $1500, and become a new member.

Then he might sit around for months or even years without working. That's why I mention, although the grass always seems greener, it isn't, until you know what you're up against on that vast lawn. Stiff competition, the best actors working in film and television and no more nonunion work, are immediate facts of life for a new member. If you're up to speed through training and ample professional experience, it may be the time to sign up, but if you aren't, stick to the nonunion stuff for awhile longer. In LA, you can actually make a living as a nonunion performer.

Entry to SAG is an important goal for all professional actors in Hollywood and it can be a huge step for you, but it is not a panacea. Nonunion thespians should remain so as long as they can, doing as much nonunion work as they can find. They're building a serious resume and ultimately becoming finely tuned actors who can soon compete with SAG talent.

And that's another reason for not joining SAG too soon. You don't have to. As you'll find, nonunion actors, especially younger ones and those seeking opportunities in commercials, can sometimes audition for projects that fall under SAG's jurisdiction. An agent will submit and a casting director will read the right actor even if he's not in SAG. It doesn't happen on every project or to every nonunion performer, but it happens. You wouldn't base a career on this, but you can get one started.

K

Keeping the Faith

People inside and outside the industry will always remind you how hard it is to be an actor. It's a subject that nearly everyone seems to be an expert about. They're right, but you won't fully understand how hard it is until you've done it for years and survived some tough times. Your faith will be tested. Keeping it will see you through.

You'll probably never lose your passion for the acting. If you do, then find a different vocation. You will, however, have times when the business, or lack of business, will make you want to bang your head into a brick wall. You may do everything right for months and get nothing but heartache. As you get older, you'll see your friends and family members progressing through their nonacting careers nicely.

You'll still be in a field where you won't know what tomorrow will bring. It could be fame and riches, but it might just be a lifelong struggle. As a new actor, the idea is kind of romantic. As a year in and year out veteran, it can be contemplative or disturbing, no doubt related to the kind of year you're having. A great year will carry you, a bad one will challenge you.

One side of you might feel, rightfully so, that you've paid your dues; you've showed them you're a professional and now things should be easier. People like your work, hired you, and then you've never heard from them again. That's almost understandable to your business side, but it's still tough on the person inside.

You've really got to keep the faith when that happens. You've got to remind yourself that you have chosen a profession that is lucky to have you in it. Really. You've got to pat yourself on the back for waiting another day for something positive to happen. Put yourself back into that mind-set you had at twenty when anything was possible. It still is in acting.

L

Lateness

Lateness is not an option for someone who hopes to be an actor in Hollywood. You might be on the receiving end of lateness dozens of times in your career, but if you're tardy just once you pay for it.

Even in this city where everything seems to start a half hour late, it's imperative the actor always be there on schedule if not early. Hollywood will certainly wait for the powers that be—directors, producers, or writers, but if an actor doesn't make sure to arrive on time opportunity will surely pass.

You must make every effort to arrive pronto for auditions and under no circumstance should you be late for a call time once you've booked a job. Casting director Brian Myers agrees that lateness is a problem area for some actors: "You'd be surprised how you can alienate a producer or director who is sitting there waiting. A phone call to let us know you're running even five or ten minutes behind is a simple way to avoid that."

Nearly every casting director I spoke to for this book mentioned it as one of their pet peeves. Now you're only human, and sooner or later you're going to find yourself stuck in traffic or trying to figure out how to get from Hollywood to Studio City five minutes ago. If it happens, learn from your error.

I learned this hard and fast rule early. I've always been one of those people who prided himself on his ability to leave a place at the last minute and still arrive at my destination on time. Moving to a new city didn't do much to get me to change my ways, although new streets should have taught me better. I had an audition for a television show but wasted too much time around the house before finally heading out the door forty-five minutes before my call, which was forty-five minutes away by my calculations. An hour and fifteen minutes and two traffic jams later I arrived at the audition site to see the casting director walking down the stairs in the opposite direction from me followed by a handful of men—the producer, the director, and someone else who was employed—unlike me. I apologized profusely to the caster for my lateness, and she smiled and told me it was okay but the session was over. She also told me she'd have me back in.

Another actor, who undoubtedly arrived when he was supposed to, got the part, and that caster hasn't invited me back in the past five years. I blame no one but myself. I also haven't been late again for a single appointment.

Looks

Looks matter. If you believe that average-looking actors get as much work as handsome or gorgeous ones, then you are simply living in an alternate universe. Hollywood is a town that has built an empire around telegenic looks. There will always be more work for the stunning-looking actors because everyone, even other actors, likes to look at a great face up on the big screen.

Listen to how agent Craig Wyckoff describes the phenomena:

> They are the God Squad. That's what I call those gorgeous girls and guys that are just so unbelievable looking that you don't care whether they have any credits or not. Anybody who looks at their picture is going to bring them in just to meet them. If you are one of them, you get a lot more shots at the leads.

Obviously, there are lots of nonbeauties and average-looking humans filling the airwaves. There are also lots of scary, intimidating, and genuinely odd-looking actors who have very nice careers. That's because of the wonderful thing known as the supporting cast. The supporters are the meat and potatoes of any film and television show you see. Of course, the three or four leads on the latest "Friends" clone might be model beautiful, but those coming and going around them are the supporting actors, and producers and directors are much more open to those considered *average* looking.

By average, I don't mean uninteresting. For any actor to build a career and stand out from the thousands of performers trying to eke out a living, you'd better have some definable look. That look might be big and tough, ugly, funny, nebbishy—anything, you fill in the blank. The only look that is a tough sell in Hollywood is one that doesn't say much at all.

As Wyckoff notes, "That in-between type has to be a better actor. He usually makes it solely on his talent. He's the one that needs more credits and a body of work to show you."

Los Angeles—The Living Film Set and Beyond

Some days in the busier seasons it's hard to drive more than a few blocks without seeing one of those ubiquitous neon signs hanging from a telephone pole pointing directions to a nearby film set. They're shooting on the studio lots, on the the streets, and in many of the office build-ings, the beaches, the parks—anywhere they can get a permit and, in the low-budget world, even the permit is sometimes circumvented.

My favorite little coffee shop, located in a part of town that is nowhere near the media center, has a "Closed for Filming" sign on its door every month or so. Trust me, you've seen this place in a lot of films, most notably playing the role of a certain diner in which Samuel L. Jackson gave a stirring sermon in "Pulp Fiction." I have this vision that one day I'll sit at that familiar counter eating my usual breakfast of scrambled eggs and pancakes, but this time there'll be a camera pointing at me that is shooting an episode of a popular show.

Another coffee shop in midcity, you've seen it in countless movies, recently shut down its business and now has a sign in the window that reads "Available for Filming." Think about that for a moment; a real restaurant has closed shop, but now plays the part of itself in film and television. I'm telling you, it's wacky.

One day last year, I saw a guy standing in front of my house snap-ping pictures. My Irish rose up and I rushed out to ask him what he was up to! Was this guy trying to case my house for a ripoff? No, he was just scouting for locations for a film. For a minute I had forgotten where I was. When I told my neighbor the story, he let me know that a buddy of his had his house used for a commercial at $2000 per day. Could be a whole new business for an out-of-work actor? A month later, they were shooting the film a few blocks away. Hey, my house could have played that role!

In almost any part of town, there is sure to be a warehouse that houses props, wardrobe, special effects, and camera equipment. If you're within the confines of Hollywood proper, your eyes will be opened when you realize that one nondescript building after another plays host to sound and film facilities, acting, singing, dance, and voice-over classes. In this era of Los Angeles as not only the celluloid capital, but also as a serious theatre center, what used to be an abandoned space near downtown is likely being refurbished one of the many 99-seat the-aters that function as both performing space and showcase venue for actors to be seen. The business is everywhere.

Indeed, Los Angeles is the only city that has full office buildings in its downtown center that are just waiting to be filmed in. One floor of rooms are designed as all manner of police stations, the next a variety of distinctive hospital rooms, and the next chock full of spaces that look like the offices of a dozen different law firms.

Now, of course, LA is more than just show business. It's a new mil-lennium world-class city with all the industry, culture, and international flair you'd expect. It's one of our nation's major industrial commercial and financial centers. It used to be the center of all things aerospace, but we know where that industry went. The city is made up of every ethnic, religious, and political group you could ever imagine—all giving it a feel and look unlike any place in America, including New York City. There's culture, restaurants, nightlife, history, and all manner of things to keep you occupied for years.

Acting might be hard, but it would surely *seem* harder elsewhere. The sun shines all year, only taking a short hiatus in February so the rains can pay a visit, and then returns in time for the tail end of pilot season. Aside from perfect weather, nature is butted up right against a major metro area. There are hills and a great ocean nearby and full blown dessert and mountains just outside the city. People in LA love to brag that they can go to the beach and ski on the same day. To me, that seems like somebody has way too much on the schedule, but it's nice to realize you actually could do that if you wanted. I'm happy just making it from West LA to Burbank in time for a meeting.

Los Angeles or New York?

The first thing that many stepping-up actors ponder is that very question. These are the two central cities on the entertainment radar and both have their plusses. The traditional answer is—Los Angeles for film and television opportunities and New York if you're a student or hope for a career on the stage. The answer is traditional because it's accurate. Your ultimate decision will usually come down to which medium(s) is your primary focus.

Now I hear some of you saying, "But I want to do it all—stage, film, television, commercials, mime work." Okay, the last one I don't know, but you can do all the other stuff professionally in either place. In 2002 Los Angeles, there are tons of theatre jobs and New York has, since the 1990s, grown its film and television industry.

Yet, there is no sensible reason to move West if you plan on focusing on big theatre. Conversely, there is little rationale to spend the bucks of living in Manhattan if you are wanting to play guest star and supporting roles in television and film. Commercially it's a wash with most years' statistics suggesting fairly even ad work spread between the two cities. Industry-wise New York wins out because it has a combination of live and filmed shows, whereas LA is only about the latter.

If you want to focus on all mediums simultaneously, you'd have to give Los Angeles the edge. It's easier to get in theatre in LA. The type of theatre, however, might help you decide. There is plenty of quality, albeit non- or very low-paying stage work, but you won't be able to satisfy your artistic *and* financial needs from it. If your goal is to make a living at theatre (real contracts and huge houses), New York is the obvious route. Double that endorsement if you are focusing on musical theatre. Although the major touring shows hold auditions here a few times a year, New York is still the center of musical theatre and always will be. Nevertheless, LA edges out overall because of the abundance of 99-seat houses combined with the multiheaded monster called television and film and strong commercial numbers.

Luck

There is an undeniably an aleatoric nature to professional acting. Talk to any veteran performer and they'll share with you a story about how sheer luck intervened upon their career.

There are two very different kinds of luck. The first, and much more common, is made luck. For example, an actor who shows up at a casting office just as they were going crazy looking for an actor just like him has made his own luck. His lucky timing results in an audition and ultimately a booking. Another actor is researching a play in a bookstore and happens to meet a director he's long admired, which leads to a scheduled meeting and eventually a part in a film. Another actor rolls the dice and flies across the country only to find he's auditioned for a Broadway role that's already been cast. On his way home on the plane, he sits next to the composer of the show and by the time they've gotten their bags he's been asked to sing in an upcoming backer's production of a new musical.

Was it really luck, or was it something else? The encounters certainly speak of various levels of it, but what caused the luck in the first place? It was career hustle—made luck. Each performer was doing something proactive for their career—one was marketing himself via picture dropoffs, the second was researching a role in an industry bookstore, and the third was flying back from an audition. These actors made their own luck. Lucky people do that. Working actors do that.

Then there is the another kind of luck—the wacky kind—a fender bender in a parking lot that leads to an audition, a wrong number dialed that ends up resulting in an actor meeting a producer, or a performer volunteering at an animal shelter meeting a casting director who just so happens to need an actor like her the next morning. That's stuff that occurs maybe a couple of times in your lifetime, but no sensible person would count on sheer providence to steer their career. Do all the things you need to do to be a surviving actor and, if you get some luck along the way, consider it a nice bonus.

M

Managers

The oldest joke in show business; what's the difference between an agent and a manager? About five percent! Rim shot. Actually, there's a world of difference between the two, although those lines are commonly blurred depending on the management company and the agency with whom you're dealing. Some managers really do manage a client's career and some run their business more along the lines of talent agencies focusing primarily on submitting talent to hirers.

Actors are often in the land of confusion when it comes to managers. You'll never hear a thespian ask, do I need an agent? They always ask if they need a manager. Some aren't even sure what a manager does.

Personal managers, like talent agents, work for the actor with the goal of getting their client more employment. Whereas talent agents are licensed by the State of California and many are franchised by the unions, managers are not. They truly answer only to themselves and the actors they represent. They also charge higher commissions and can also act as producers—two reasons that have led many agents over the years to jump ship to the managing side. The one downside to management is that they cannot, according to California State Law, negotiate contracts. Only licensed agents are supposed to do that. The rule is only sometimes enforced.

Managers advise, strategize, steer, and all the while attempt to put together the big picture for your career. They are not only concerned with what you're reading for next week, but also where you'll be in one to five years down the line. It's supposed to be more, well, *personal.* They commonly earn fifteen percent commission on all the money you make so they'd better do all of that and more. This is a reason managers sometimes get a bad rap. There are indeed some who don't do much for their clients beyond collecting that commission for work the actor has either gotten themselves or through the agent's work. This annoys actors and their agents, but it angers the quality managers much more so. The fact is, most personal managers are strong contributors to their clients' successes, but you don't hear too much about those cases, only about the ones who don't work out.

Los Angeles personal manager Phil Brock founded his company, Studio Talent Group, seven years ago, and he is also the Director emeritus of the Talent Managers Association (formerly the Conference of Personal Managers), a collective of personal managers that banded together to provide their industry with common ethics and standards and also to establish the rates managers would charge. Explains Brock:

> It's fifteen percent instead of ten percent (agent's standard commission). Hopefully what you're paying that extra five percent for is the time involved. You're paying a manager for his expertise in helping to work with you on training, photographs, marketing, on innovative ideas and to make your career much more productive than it might be otherwise.

A good manager shouldn't have too many clients and can therefore devote significant time to each client, whereas many talent agencies, with a multitude of clients, just don't have much more time for things other than submitting and negotiating contracts. Here's where the lines blur a bit. Some agents, and not just the stars' ones either, do those managerial things and have all aspects of their actor's professional careers covered. In such a case, an actor would probably have no need for a manager.

Or would he?

What about a manager who has solid industry contacts and perhaps knows more casting directors' direct phone numbers than your very caring talent agent? How about one of the big ones who are able to actually produce the show? In both of those cases, a manager would make complete sense.

Fueling the negative comments you'll occasionally hear about managers are things like, "They're not licensed, so watch out," or "They're not necessary." And that last one even comes from agents and even casting directors on occasion. On the other side, there are very successful actors, some stars, who have only a manager, no agent, and are exceedingly happy with the arrangement. It's no wonder actors are really confused by the whole manager thing.

Do you need a manager? It depends. In the past, common wisdom was that you had a manager when you were working so much that you literally needed someone to coordinate all your activity while planning for the jobs ahead. Rarely would an actor who wasn't employed regularly have much use for a personal manager.

That's not necessarily the case now. With so many actors, and many of them union performers, unable to find an agent (seventy-five percent of SAG members are without an agent), a manager might be the way to go. Although they cannot legally negotiate a contract in California without an agent, as they can in much of the rest of the country, managers can do pretty much everything else and ultimately help that actor find an agent, too.

Given the similarity in what they do, you would think agents and managers would get along better overall, but in many cases they just can't get past the divide that has existed between the two parties for years. When it works, everyone benefits, and the actor has two sets of eyes and ears looking out for her, but when egos and competition gets in the way, there can be waves.

"I don't think it should be adversarial," says Brock. "I will tell you there are a couple of agents in town that I know of who aren't happy if their clients look to gain a manager. My theory on that is that is it's because they haven't been doing their job successfully as an agent and they're fearful that the manager is going to come and automatically remove the client. I don't do that. My job is to come in and add to the mix."

I know Brock's statement is pretty accurate because I saw it first-hand when I worked at a talent agency in New York City in the early 1990s. In most cases, the agents got along and worked in tandem with managers. On occasion, a manager would get too aggressive or try to shake things up and the feathers would fly, but that was rare. Generally, when a manager was calling it was because the actor wasn't getting out and that checks and balances was a pretty fair system for keeping an actor as a priority.

Marketing

If you want to succeed in Hollywood you can't sit around and be the misunderstood starving artist waiting to be discovered. You've got to hustle to make a living and find repeat opportunities to do so. No one is going to take you under their wing. There are too many actors in Hollywood who have the looks, talent, drive, *and* the marketing savvy required to be a working actor.

How do you market? To whom do you market? How often should you market? Like everything else in show business, there is no scientific equation—only common methods that have proven effective. You can use these familiar marketing techniques and skew them to your unique methodology.

Most actors live and breathe by mailed submissions in Los Angeles. It's not like New York, where you make the daily rounds. Here, if you're in a certain area or auditioning at a particular studio, you might drop a picture, but generally you'll be relying on the postal service in this city to be your go-to partner in marketing.

The big marketing question is whether you believe in the effort and expense of mass mailings. Mass mailings are defined slightly differently by everyone, but they encompass sending potentially hundreds of headshots, postcards, or flyers in one giant effort. Some actors believe in mass mailings; others are skeptical of the expense–return ratio. I've done mass mailings and believe they work, but experience has taught me that they are best employed in rare occasions. I'm comfortable suggesting that a true mass mailing, meaning one that finds the desk of most casting directors, agents, ad agencies, and perhaps some producers is best used for your first contact only. A new actor to Los Angeles owes it to himself to do a big kick-off, if only to set the foundation for future contact.

Even without that huge hit all at once, there are still the hundreds of casting contacts and agency names to consider. Who do you choose? Savvy veterans learn how to pare the list down to workable numbers— focused mailings, if you will. They identify the casting directors who are the busiest and hire their type, and then market primarily to them. They send pictures to the agencies that represent talent at a similar skill and credit level. They sometimes mail to the directors and producers of programs who they can see themselves being hired by and even better to those by whom they've been formerly employed. Spending some time on research and speaking to your fellow actors will help you to find the people most likely to use your services.

Once you've established your chosen contacts, mailings are done whenever there is something of substance to announce. It might be a stage play in which you are appearing, an announcement of a booking or appearance on a television show or in a film, or for lack of work, a few plugs about some auditions or callbacks you've recently had. It can be anything that puts your face in front of them, along with a positive and career-forwarding piece of news.

In the absence of real news, actors have their own theories about how many marketing mailings to take on. Because there is no universally accepted number, most rely on their gut instinct to guide them. Generally, every two to three months is appropriate to each party unless you have some major news to announce. Major news almost always means a booking or an upcoming appearance.

Once you've covered your A list, you also want to branch out and send submissions to some new people whom you haven't met yet. It's always good to expand your marketing horizons lest you become too reliant on the people who have formerly read you or hired you. That's a sure way to extended unemployment.

Here are the most popular forms of marketing for the working actor:

- *Headshot Mailings*—This is by far the most well-known method used by new and veteran actors alike. For initial contacts, in particular, there is no better way to introduce yourself to casting directors, agents, and, to a lesser extent, directors and producers. Whether you are doing a single picture, a series of minimailings (perhaps five to twenty sent at a time), or a mass mailing (anywhere from several dozen to several hundred) in one fell swoop, headshot mailings have proven an effective method for getting your face in front of people.

  Lists of all the potential mailing recipients are available at local bookstores, and actors must avail themselves of only the most-updated lists possible. Headshots are expensive to mail. At a current $.60 a piece, you will be throwing your money away if you are sending to people that have moved from an old address. Don't count on mail forwarding—the caster may be three offices removed by that time. Casting directors are always in new offices, agents move from one company to another, and producers and directors have a new home every time they start a new film or television show. Only a small population have permanent addresses, so make sure you do your research before attempting any mailing.

  Aside from that first contact, headshots mailings are best used when you are submitting for a specific role on a project. You'll choose the headshot that represents appearancewise the role you are seeking. All submissions, whatever the contact reason, should include a short cover letter detailing the reason for the mailing. It could be "submitting for the project," "introducing myself to you," and so on, as long as it looks professional and respects the time of the person looking at it. Keep it short. If you have been personally recommended by someone in the party to whom you are sending the headshot, make sure you note that at the top of the letter.

  Headshots are also sent by experienced performers whenever they have a new picture or whenever their resume has changed dramatically since a past last mailing.

  A key thing to remember with headshot marketing is to know to whom you're sending. A smiling commercial shot would probably be wasted on a casting director who is busy hiring tough, menacing, or urban types for a one-hour drama. Conversely, your picture featuring your best serious look would be wasted if sent to a sitcom caster. With an agent, it's always your best picture right now, not the one you are thinking of using in the future.

  Actors often ask whether they should submit headshots to casting directors if they already have an agent. The answer is, "ask your agent." I've never known one who didn't want timely mailings from the talent to casters. Timely is the key. Weekly or even monthly mailings might just serve to annoy and make your rep's job harder. Talk to your agent or manager and work out a plan. Some may not mind a general submission every few months but don't want you to submit for specific shows or roles.

- *Postcards* —In an industry where your face is your calling card, you need to get that card seen by many. For general submissions, sending 8×10s to industry contacts who already know you is an expensive and unnecessary thing to do thanks to the wonderful 4×6 postcard, essentially a smaller version of your headshot. Actors in all parts of the country use them, but Los Angeles performers rely on them as a way to stay in touch with the hundreds of casting directors in the city. I'm a big believer in postcards as the most effective and economical method of marketing.

If you crunch the numbers, you'll find that an annual budget for mailing can be quite tough on the average surviving actor. Add up the postage, envelopes, resume costs, and running off numerous lithographs and you'll realize this isn't a nickel-and-dime affair.

In April 2002, I priced out the following to give you a better idea of the cost factor. Let's base this on a very conservative number of 500 headshots versus 500 postcards. First, let's look at the cost of reproducing. I spoke with three of the busier printing houses in LA, and the average cost of five hundred 8×10s is $102. (You'll always buy in bulk because the price drops substantially.) The average cost of five hundred postcards is $88. That's not a huge difference, but when you factor it over many years it adds up. The big difference, however, comes in the cost of mailing. The mailing cost for five hundred 8×10s is currently $300 (at $.60 per picture). The cost of mailing the same amount of postcards is $115 (at $.23 per postcard). That's a staggering sixty-two percent savings.

The key for the surviving actor is to not waste the mailing. How effective is simply sending a postcard with a message such as, "Please remember I'm out here." It's certainly better than doing nothing, and you'd have to guess that an actor doing that once or twice a year is going to have better success than one who doesn't market himself in any fashion.

You're spending hard-earned money to do these mailings, and you'd be a lot happier if you used that blank space to the left of the person's name to tell them something of substance. By Hollywood survival standards, here is the descending order of importance:

1. *Announce that you are appearing in something.* For instance, say, "Hello. I'll be appearing in the 10/24 episode of 'Mike's House' as the insurance salesman on ABC at 9:00," or something like,

"I'll be performing as Biff in the Omega Theatre production of 'Death of a Salesman' from August 15 through October 10. Please contact me for complimentary tickets."

The information on both postcards was substantial and specific. Each actor let the recipient know the role, time or location, and dates. Don't assume the person is going to know you or be willing to look up when or where a show is airing or being performed. Keep your postcards short and informative.

Send them to casting directors and agencies, too, if you are looking for new representation. Other mailings could be to directors and producers whom you know or with whom you have worked or hope to work with, but you'll have your work cut out for you getting current addresses for those people. You do not write, "I'll be appearing with my friend Nick in a video we're shooting in my living room." You're a professional and as such should only announce professional credits, not home movies.

What do you put if you haven't worked recently or don't have a performance to endorse? Assuming it's been awhile since you did a mailing, at least a couple of months, you might consider the following.

2. *Promote a significant achievement short of an actual job.* Even non-bookings can be a positive career statement. For example, say, "Hello. I had recent callbacks for Burger King and Hasbro. I was also put on avail for Pacific Bell," or, "Recently had second callback for national touring company of 'The Producers.'"

Callbacks and on avails reflect talent, momentum, and progress, and are good stuff for a postcard or even headshot mailing. The flip side is not to overpromote nonbookings. On the surface, "I've had fifty commercial auditions in three months" might sound impressive, but you risk the reader wondering why you haven't booked any of them.

3. *Announce positive growth in your abilities or industry progress.* For example, "Hello. I've just been accepted into Harry Lipscomb's advance on-camera class and recently joined SAG. I'd welcome the opportunity to read for you."

It's not "set the world on fire" news, but you're telling industry people that you are being proactive in the advancement of your career, and that's a smart thing to plug. There are other reasons to promote via postcard, and a common motive is for to let them know you are reachable differently than in the past.

4. *Change of representation and contact numbers.* For example, "Please note that I am now signed with the Betty Berman Talent Group for theatrical representation." If no agent is currently in your life, you might just explain, "New contact number is 310-555-5555."

Something that's become very popular, especially on postcards that have only a line of information, is for the actor to print a miniresume on the postcard back. This is a way of showing credits and picture without the expense of an 8×10 mailing. They can be effective, as long as the type is clear and large enough to read. However, they are a distant second to mailing the 8×10 with full-size resume for first contact.

Speaking of type, unless you have impeccable penmanship, you are better off printing your information on labels or directly onto the postcard, if your printer accepts postcards. It's cleaner and more professional looking. That'll add a few cents onto the budget, but what you gain in appearance is often worth the cost.

Between headshots and postcards, you'll be able to cover a large amount of your day-to-day marketing needs, but there are some other methods that can also help your cause.

- *Trade Notices*—It is not uncommon for an actor to take out a small ad in a trade paper (*Variety, Hollywood Reporter*) when they are appearing in a nice-size role. The expense of such a promo can approach mass mailing rates, but you will be hitting a large segment of the industry on the day your show might be airing. Such efforts should always be coordinated so that the ad, with a picture of yourself, comes out on the morning of, or the day before, an airing. It works twofold. It announces your airtime, and even if people don't tune in to see you, and they usually won't, they'll see that you are working. Hollywood loves a winner, so it could bode well to go this route.

  But don't overdo it. One young actor took out ads week after week in a trade paper announcing that he was in a new class or that he'd just had a great audition. That's not the way to go. Even when what you have to announce is genuine, you wouldn't do this more than a few times in your career or you risk appearing an egoist. There's a fine line between smart marketing and self-flagellation.

  But don't think a little self-promotion isn't acceptable. You've seen those ads for actors announcing *For Your Consideration,* in regard to trying to get an actor nominated for some award or another. Sometimes the studios pay for them, other times the agencies pay for them, and often the actors pay for them themselves.

- *Invites and Flyers*—A much better and more common way to market is through show invitations. Again, the objective is to remind someone of your existence, and they have a lot of actors to be reminded of, so what better way than if you are acting in show. You'll send a flyer to the person in mind a couple of weeks before the production begins and then possibly follow up within a few days of the performance. Follow-ups are usually done when you know the person well enough to phone their office. The flyer will have the show dates and a contact number to call for complimentary tickets. It's hard to get industry people to come out, so when they do agree to a show the onus is on you to make sure those tickets are waiting for them at the box office.

- *Drop-Offs*—Drop-offs are a surefire way to run your engine into the ground if you don't approach them sensibly. Los Angeles is just too immense to get out and drive around for hand deliveries more than a couple of times per month. That doesn't mean you can't organize a plan for logical drop-offs that works with your ever-changing schedule. When times are good, you will find yourself getting auditions from one end of town to the other. Always keep a box of headshots and updated resumes in your trunk for when you're in a certain part of town or on a particular studio lot. When in an area, you can choose two or three people with whom you want to try and meet or perhaps remind you're out there by hand delivering a picture to their office. Drop-offs are not encouraged or discouraged, but you have to respect that you are visiting their space without an appointment. That means you come in, drop the picture off, say hello if there is someone in the lobby to say hello to, and then get out of there. If you barge in as if you are expected, you will ruffle feathers. Do it the right way, and you might even land an unexpected audition every once in awhile.

- *Phone Calls*—Phone calls to casting directors are a subject that causes the hair on your arms to stand on end. Actors fear making phone calls to casting offices for good reason. The people on the other end usually don't want to hear from you. To that end, I suggest to only consider a call to someone with whom you have a professional relationship that warrants it. What warrants it? The only time you are going to get away with phone calls if it's to someone you have worked for several times, someone who knows you well, likes your presence, and most of all someone who has previously told you that you may check in via phone from time to time. You'll have maybe a few of those in your career. Don't take it for granted that because someone has hired you that they want you to phone them in the future. That's not the way it works. The rule of thumb with casting directors and phone calls, in general, is that you call them when you're returning their phone call. As far as staying in contact with your own agent, this is also a form of marketing and is something you'll definitely need to do. How often and during which business hours (excluding emergency calls) is a subject you'll discuss with your talent representative upon signing your contract. You have to remember that an agency has many clients and a friendly marketing maneuver to them might be called for from time to time.

- *Demo Reels*—Demos are expensive to duplicate and mail, and you'll only market with them on the occasion that someone requests seeing it. Do not mail your demo out unsolicited. It will probably not be seen. In your cover letter, which you'll send with your headshot, you will mention that you have video demo and would be glad to supply it upon request. When you're contacted and told to do so, send or drop off your reel as soon as possible. Always include a self-addressed, stamped envelope for return of the reel. It's a lot cheaper than making more copies.

N

Neighborhoods

Where to live, where to live? Los Angeles presents that question at each freeway off-ramp. As a surviving actor, your goal is pretty basic—you must be near enough to everything that is related to the business. Unfortunately, everything doesn't cooperate. The entertainment industry is spread over hundreds of square miles from the Westside, to the Valley, and east to downtown—it's everywhere and anywhere, and occasionally it's even in Hollywood proper.

There are literally fifty great parts of town where you could live and about a thousand different streets with great apartments, so I'm not telling you where to find a place, but I do have some thoughts on practical convenience.

For your first place, I'd suggest this proposal; live within a fifteen-minute drive (nonrush hour) of the Hollywood Hills, perhaps as far west as Bundy and as far east as Vermont, as far south as Washington, as far north as Burbank Boulevard. That will cover about ninety percent of your auditioning, training, and living needs. Within that range, you can find many affordable areas with good housing in all budgets.

This location works on many levels, not the least of which is the amount of daily driving you'll be doing. A bizarre fact of the business is that wherever you live will still seem to be the furthest distance from where you'll need to be for most of your acting stuff. It's just one of those things. If you live in the Valley in Studio City, a perfectly sensible spot for an actor to reside given the heavy industry presence there, you'll find yourself landing auditions mostly on the other side of the hill. Your agent will be on the Westside. Conversely, if you move closer to Westside, the casting directors who have offices in the Valley will finally start calling you. It's screwy, but you'll still be very happy that you're getting auditions. In the end, no matter what you do, you're going to get stuck behind the wheel a lot. Residing in or near that hill zone helps you to cut down the mileage overall. Driving less means more study time and less expense. The downside is that there'll be fewer chances for you to see billboard legend Angelyne tooling around in her pink Corvette.

While preparing this book, I was also in the process of selling my house (no reflection on how well I thought the book would sell) and went apartment hunting for the first time in four years. My wife and I canvassed the whole city—from Tarzana to Los Feliz, from Santa Monica to Burbank. I've seen things you don't want to see. Take it from me and observe these simple rules. When an apartment manager tells you that the apartment is charming, quaint, or homey, they mean it is very small. If they tell you the neighborhood is eclectic, funky, or edgy, they usually mean the crime statistics are enormous. If they say they don't have an agent and would like to meet yours in exchange for a rent reduction, find another building quickly.

Actually you will find many actors managing apartment buildings, but I doubt any would ask for your agent's name. They will, however, show you some pretty amazing spaces. If you're coming here from New York City, as so many performers do, you'll think you are in heaven. Apartments are absolutely huge compared with Manhattan. In fact, some cars are huge compared with Manhattan apartments. However, those from New York, San Francisco, or Tokyo will find Los Angeles rental prices very reasonable; if you're from anywhere else, they'll seem high. There are a wide variety of accommodations available from cozy (that's yet another word for small) singles to spacious apartments with balconies or terraces, to luxury townhomes with all the amenities, to detached single-family homes with full yards.

Some neighborhoods split off from their historical names to separate themselves from higher crime areas that may be right nearby. If you have any doubt about a neighborhood, call the local police department and ask to speak to the lead officer. With some prodding and a promise that you aren't with a newspaper, they will usually share crime statistics for their jurisdiction. They used to offer that information openly, but realtors in sketchier areas started threatening lawsuits. Overall, though, most areas of LA where actors congregate are safe.

Once you've found a few places that you can afford, even if you don't have a survival job for a month or two, I suggest you call your car insurance company. Prices can be dramatically different from one part of town to the next. You may find your cheap apartment isn't so cheap when they're going to jack your insurance rate twenty percent higher. Maybe the other apartment just a mile away for $25 more per month will mean much better car insurance rates and ultimately less overall expenditures per month.

In no particular order, here are just a few areas that are actor friendly, affordable, and safe: Sherman Oaks, Studio City, Burbank, Mid-Wilshire, and West LA near Olympic or Pico. There are many other communities that are great, too.

People have written to me at *Backstage West* wondering what Hollywood is all about. Here's the deal as I see it. Hollywood is in the middle of major gentrification right now. It's a lot nicer and safer than it's been in the past, and it's undeniably centrally located. There are some rough areas and some nicer residential areas to the famous namesake. However, I still don't recommend it for a new arrival to the city. You'll probably settle-in better in a quieter, less hectic environment. After a few years, you can move again once you know the city better.

There are apartment and house listings in the *Los Angeles Times* every Sunday. Web sites are also growing increasingly popular as a way to help people find rentals. With neighborhood descriptions and photos that can save you a lot of time and gasoline, I suggest you spend a few hours on the Internet. One I've used twice with success is westsiderentals.com. There are also roommate services available if you have the burning desire to live with another actor.

There are also more expensive areas that you can consider, such as Brentwood, Beverly Hills, Santa Monica, West Hollywood, and Century City, but the rents there are high. Unless you are financially set or have a few working roommates, you don't need to rent in those areas when starting out in LA.

Many people associate Los Angeles with the beach and the ocean. They're definitely here, but if you want to live near them you'll pay through the nose. Because there are only a few entertainment entities in that area, you'll be doing plenty of cross-town driving. If extra driving and high rents aren't a concern, you can consider Santa Monica, Venice, and maybe even south to Marina Del Rey.

Nepotism

Nepotism is rampant in Hollywood. It's hard to look through a cast list of more than two or three shows without finding at least a few names of those related to more famous individuals sharing the same family name. Then there are all the famous sons, daughters, nephews, and nieces of the well known who take on different last names to distance themselves for the image of their A-list relative, at least to a degree. They want the public to give them their fair due, but it's certainly okay if people in the industry know they're related to a power player.

Show business is fond of hiring within the family. And not just actors either, although they certainly get the most attention and seem to have the most to prove to a scrutinizing public. Aside from actors, cameramen, grips, set designers, stunt men, directors, and writers, all spawn offspring or support other relatives who take up the family trade. Why shouldn't they?

Nepotism is as much American as is apple pie. Doctors in Detroit want their kids to be doctors. Firemen in Fresno want their kids to be firemen. Why then wouldn't a famous Hollywood actor or producer want their kids to follow in their footsteps? It's no different.

Yet, people love to grouse when a famous producer's daughter decides she wants to act or when a casting director's son starts showing up in his mom's projects. The loudest complaints come from the nonconnected actors who believe they are competing for, or rather not getting a chance to compete for, work with the blessed rung jumpers.

However, it hardly matters that there is nepotism in this business. The truth is that, when you're focused on not getting work, you look for reasons to complain. Nepotism is just one of the easier targets, but it won't affect your career. No number of daughters and sons of the elite are going to keep you from having a wonderful career.

Besides, try to put yourself in that person's shoes for just a minute. How many eyes are on them each time they try to do anything? A lot of people are just waiting for them to fall, because they share a last name with someone famous. Give them a break and let them try to achieve their dream just as you are. So what if they made it with some help? Who doesn't need help in this world? And then remember this, too. When you've succeeded in your career and have a house in the hills and the satisfaction of having made it in one of the world's toughest careers, maybe you'll start a family and one day one of those kids might say, "Mommy, I wanna be an actor." I have the sneaky suspicion that you'll help the kid out.

Nonunion Work

True: You'll have a much better chance to have a long career as an actor in Los Angeles if you are a SAG member.

False: You cannot audition or do union work without a union card.

True: Franchised agencies are more inclined to work with union actors.

False: Agents won't work with nonunion actors because they can't get them auditions for the union projects.

Let's put this to rest once and for all. Of course, you'll want to be in SAG when you are eligible, but you needn't be a member to be employed in one of their films. So many young actors rush to Hollywood and freak out because they are under the impression that no one will work with them as a nonunion actor. That's false, too, for a few reasons.

Here again are the two words every nonunion actor should know—Taft–Hartley. Remember, this means that a nonunion performer can audition for SAG fare and actually perform in a union film, show, or commercial for a work period of up to thirty days.

There's another big reason you needn't be alarmed if you're not in SAG. Los Angeles has a ton of nonunion acting work. This may be the only place in America where one can actually make a monetary living as a nonunion actor. Even within LA's nonunion ranks, there are some very seasoned performers, so don't think getting this work will be any easier than it is in the union world. Although the goal for most is to hurriedly get that SAG card, there are others who are too just busy working to be concerned.

Nonunion includes everything from student films—which may or may not ultimately come through with your payment, in this case, a video copy of your work—all the way up to large projects that resemble union shoots right down to the budgets and what they pay the talent. As you build credits and move up the nonunion ladder, you'll improve your skills and search for jobs that not only afford you the opportunity to perform, but also help you to afford to pay your rent—in other words, gigs that come with a paycheck.

Casting director Tina Seiler explains some of the type of shows where a nonunioner might find work:

> There are many nonunion opportunities such as student and independent films, industrials and reality reenactment shows. While I cast many union projects, I have also cast several nonunion reenactment shows. These shows are usually nonunion due to the many people that are used in each reenactment, sometimes as many as fifteen to twenty.

The key to nonunion survival is knowing when to say "no," and it changes over time. You have to decide which nonunion job is right for you at each stage of your career. Is it simply a performance outlet to get experience in front of a camera? Fine, great, take anything offered if you'd like. Or maybe you're past that and are seeking higher-quality projects that will showcase you in more substantial roles? At that point you say "yes" only to those kinds of offers. Eventually, you'll move to the next level and only accept professional roles that also will compensate you monetarily. Then you may consider only those that pay a certain amount. It's a step-by-step process, and everyone has their own pace. Sooner or later, to reach the studio and major network jobs, you will have to say "no" altogether to nonunion work and step up to AFTRA and SAG.

Nonunion, being the wide open market that it is, has every type of remuneration imaginable. Producers of nonunion films, shows, music videos, and industrials know that they have access to top talent who will work for much less than union performers. So it's not uncommon for projects to pay $50 to a $100 per day for principal talent. Others, though, want only the best and most experienced actors and are willing to pay for it. Some nonunion jobs pay into the thousands for extended shoots, and it's not uncommon for a nonunion dayplayer to get close to SAG scale for a commercial or film role if the project has a real budget. Some wonder why a producer who has real money would ever go nonunion. A few reasons of many are; no future residual payments, no pension and health payments, and no one to tell him how many hours he can work his actors without paying them more. They save a lot of money in the end and can get away with a lot more—all the more reason for a nonunion performer to pick and choose his projects carefully.

Tina Seiler adds this on the payday factor:

> Many companies doing industrials have a small budget and therefore are nonunion. Sometimes they pay well and sometimes it is just for a copy. In doing low budget films and student films you should be aware that you are doing this mostly for the experience, copy and to be able to put a film on your resume. You will probably never get the deferred pay they tell you about.

Seiler is right. Deferred payment to most knowledgeable actors means no payment. As far as student films are concerned, the only promise of payment will be the video copy of your work, but even that is hard to get. I've had countless letters sent to *Backstage West* from frustrated actors who have hounded student filmmakers to get a copy of the project or at least their scenes. I've even contacted the deans of the various film schools to alert them to this growing problem. To date, only one, the Dean of the UCLA film school has responded, promising to remind his students of their obligation to professional actors, whether they are nonunion or union.

You can rest assured that, by sticking to the projects that do pay, that are produced by reputable companies, and that are cast by established casting directors, you'll probably get your payment without any hassle. Aside from experience, a credit, and payment, Seiler notes another reason nonunion fare can be a boon to a fledgling career: "Keep in mind, that on any of these projects, if the producer, director or CD like you, they will probably use you again on another project of theirs, which might be on a much larger scale."

Some nonunion environments will be hardly distinguishable from low-budget SAG sets. You'll work with talented casts, top notch crews, and ace directors, and there'll be nice budgets, too. Be thankful for those. Others won't be so attractive, confusion reigns, and they expect you to work for sixteen hours with three hours off before your next call while sitting outside freezing between shots. Some will have fully functional soundstages at their disposal and great food during meal breaks, others will be taping in barren wildernesses without ample lighting and a bag of carrots being passed around as your first meal of the day, twelve hours from when you began.

There is nothing wrong with checking out a prospective employer. Some nonunion production companies and producers have exemplary track records. Others do not. Do your research, because there isn't a union to back you up if things go astray. Nonunion actors are more or less their own union. If there is a problem with a working condition or a payment issue, you might have to fight the battle yourself. Of course, there is the Department of Consumer Affairs, the Los Angeles court system, and other agencies that could come to your aid.

Nonunion jobs can be found in *Backstage West* and in small numbers on Breakdown Service's free Actor Access area at www.breakdownservices.com/access/awindex.htm. Many of the larger budgeted nonunion gigs end up on the other Breakdowns, which actors are not allowed to view. These jobs are cast through one of the many casting directors in town that specialize in nonunion projects. Your chances of ending up on a good shoot and being paid what you were promised increase when you seek those projects cast by the top nonunion people. It won't take you more than a few weeks in Los Angeles to learn who's who in the casting world.

As a smart nonunion actor, you'll learn which casters are the busiest and most highly regarded in the nonunion realm. You'll market to them. You'll also hear the names of respected production companies that do top-quality nonunion jobs. Those are the ones for whom you'll strive to work. If you play your cards smart, you can do years of nonunion work in this market and work on some really good projects, while drawing a decent paycheck every once in awhile.

On more than a few occasions, you will submit to a company you don't know. Most will be fine, but you'll find a couple that will be unprofessional. As soon as you get a whiff of ineptitude, and you'll know it when you smell it, head the other direction. If you sense a scam, and they tend to show up more often in the nonunion world, run even faster.

Agents, even franchised ones, will commonly charge nonunion actors twenty percent to negotiate nonunion contracts. That's twice as much as in the union world, but having a talent representative deal with the producer is a good measure of protection. Many actors, however, choose to take care of business themselves at this level. If you're one of them, check contracts closely for payment, hours, and responsibilities. If there isn't a formal contract offered, you have every right to ask for deal memo of some type to confirm the agreement before the shoot date. You can also ask nothing other than where to show up for work, but there's a risk to that. You may be told the contract will be signed on–set; however, try to see it and sign it beforehand. If you don't, make sure you do before you step in front of the camera for the first time. I heard from one actress who was strung along all day with the promise of "it's on the way." She and her fellow actors worked all day, were wrapped without ever having gotten their contracts, and never saw a dime of their payment.

Nudity

At some point in your career, you may be asked to disrobe for a scene in a film or television show. If you look like a caveman, you will probably keep your clothes on throughout. However, if you fit the demographic of the attractive female between eighteen and twenty-eight, sooner or later a part you'll read for will include nudity.

Should you do it? First, on the "don't" side. If you refuse, your career won't end before it starts. There may be a few out there who still insist you have to drop your blouse and maybe even skirt on-camera if you want to make it as a starlet, but those few are on the way out little by little. You don't have to do it. However, it could cost you a role along the way. Can you live without a job or two? Of course you can. When you're famous, you can get a body double like many well-known actresses do.

Second, for the "go ahead and do it" side. The movie-going public does like to see a little skin, let's be honest. If it's your skin and you agree to do it, you'll be pleased to know that there are cameramen and makeup people, and oftentimes sensitive directors, who can make the experience much less painful.

If you're comfortable with your body and being nude in front of strangers doesn't intimidate you, then being willing to take it off might even get you a job or two. Just be cautious. If the role is a legitimate one and there's some nudity, it's one thing. If the part is just about nudity and the role is nothing more than a showcase for your body, then you may be getting into a situation that isn't going to do anything for a serious career. Pick and choose these situations carefully. It's one thing if someone asks you to take off your top for a beach scene in a studio blockbuster. If it's a guy with a camera in his living room and he wants to improv, you'd better stay away. Some attractive actresses make a career around their physical attributes. If you're content doing B movies or soft erotica (you see them on cable late at night, usually a semblance of a story line involving a handsome detective, a great house in the Hollywood Hills, and lots of nude women), there are legitimate opportunities in that genre as well. Again, pick carefully and think about your bigger career plan. And, yes, this also goes for men. The ubiquitous butt shot has become the norm.

A soundstage full of semistaring people will make the sturdiest actor freak, but many sets are closed when these scenes are shot. If yours isn't, you can demand that it be so. All this is discussed upfront well before the shoot day. If you get to the set and things don't seem right, keep your clothes on. Remember, you are the one that must always be looking out for you.

If a director really wants you for a part and you are averse to playing nudity, you can still work things out. Stars do it all the time and so do nonstars who are the director's first choice. The wonderful solution to this dilemma is a body double.

They are usually perfect physical specimens who are glad to take it all off or play any individual part of your physique—private areas and all. You won't be disappointed, as these actresses and actors have great figures and that'll only make you look all the better.

Obviously, all this has to do with on-camera nudity. You should not appear nude at auditions. If someone ever tells you should get nude for them in private to advance your career, steer them to the nearest strip club and go on your way.

Numbers

Acting is a numbers game for many reasons. The combined national membership of SAG and AFTRA is around 190,000. Add in another 45,000 Actor's Equity members working stages across the United States. Then there are the nonunion actors whose numbers easily eclipse the total in all the unions. There are also the sometime actors who have other careers but occasionally do professional performance work. There are community theatre actors, student actors, professional sports and music stars who occasionally try to emote, and the scourge of the industry—the real people, who are sometimes used, primarily in commercials, for their *realness.*

For such a niche profession, there are certainly a lot of people doing it to one degree or another. You can't let yourself get lost in those numbers and it's easy enough to do when you become aware that there will never be enough work to go around. That's the second set of numbers you must accept as a reality. There aren't that many roles available, and they often go to a fairly small fraction of the acting community. You can break into the professional, but it's tough work. You must maximize your opportunities to remain there for any length of time. Even on the best day, the amount of work will never come close to the amount of talent vying to get it.

As casting director Lisa Miller Katz notes, "There are so many good actors out there that I just can't hire. I have one or two roles on *Everybody*

Loves Raymond each week and I get thousands of pictures. I mean, you have to do the math. There's just not that much work out there."

To get that work, you'll also need to audition a good number of times. In television and films, you will read for many things that you won't book. That's the nature of the beast. But to survive, you'll have to keep the ratio to a reasonable number. You must get callbacks and eventually book some work if you're going to last in the professional ranks. For commercials, you might read for fifty projects and not get one of them. This wouldn't be practical for television shows or films. All you can do is make each one count as much as possible. Prepare well and your numbers will come.

Even if you do land a part, the money you'll make is something you must face as a professional. Due to salary contraction, many working-class actors are making less than they have in the past. If an actor gets his quote rate she's usually very happy, but many are forced to work for less than they are accustomed. If you aren't making much more than union scale and are only booking a few jobs a year, you could find it very difficult to survive show business. Building up to larger parts, which, in turn, leads to better paychecks, is the method most actors hope to use to overcome this number reality. However, survival jobs and living modestly are other ways to help you in this regard.

Finally, how you market yourself numberwise can greatly affect how you'll do in the acting field over the long haul. Treat yourself like the business person that you are, which means regular promotion. Many actors who stand out from the crowd are not only focused and talented but also remember most of show business *is* business. As such, they market with consistent mailings.

As manager Phil Brock reveals,

> If there were five identical actors, I want the one who is going to be passionate about what they do, who is going to be devoted to find ways to sell themselves better and market themselves better every day. I don't want the actor who is going to sit at home and bemoan his fate. I want the actor who gets up every morning and says, "Where's my audition?" "What else can I do for my career?"

O

On-Set

Regardless of what type of shoot you're working on, there is one survival tool that must be employed from the minute you arrive on the set until the time you leave—common sense. There hasn't been a guidebook written on how to behave on every set. Few casting directors or agents have the time to tell you, nor could they possibly spell out the multitude of situations that might occur. Thus, you must use good old common sense to get you through the work day.

Every set is different. Some are run like military operations, whereas others are laid back and carefree. Some treat actors, especially the extras, like cattle, whereas others embrace all the talent like they're part of the family. Some sets refuse to let anyone but the stars roam around, and others let everyone do their own thing. You might find smiling faces, have access to a free telephone, and discover good snacks one day, but find just the opposite on the same set the next day.

In short, you must be able to readily adapt to what each new day brings. It's not brain surgery, however, if you do the right things and have a flexible personality, your day on a set should be enjoyable, educational, occasionally inspiring, and, ultimately, profitable.

First, you've got to get there. Studio lots are especially notorious in the early hours for busy traffic, so get an early start when commuting. You might not find any traffic on the highway at that hour, but you're bound to encounter a long line of cars waiting to get through lot security. Since September 11, studio lots have taken on a fortress mentality at the front gates. There continues to be serious concern by American media companies regarding threats, and Hollywood has smartly decided to not take any chances. Consequently, wait times are much longer than they were previously. Add an extra half hour and you'll be fine. Do not forget your driver's license, or you may never get past the gate.

Check in with the studio guard, give them the name of the production on which you'll be working, and they'll supply you with a lot pass and a parking assignment. Don't be surprised if your parking spot is at the furthest possible point away from the sound stage on which you're shooting. The good spaces are reserved for stars and studio executives, so it's not a good career move to take Mr. Eisner's parking space. Because you'll probably be walking a good distance, wear a comfortable pair of shoes and plan on an extra fifteen-minute hike from your car to the check-in area. Some studios have shuttle vans that run from outlying parking areas to the back lots and sound stages, but you're more than likely to find these only sporadically. Off-lot location shooting is less formalized, so if you arrive early enough you might have just as good a chance to park as close to the set as a name performer. On bigger shoots off the lots, you'll often have to park in crew parking that could be a block or a mile from the actual set. There'll usually be a security guard who'll direct you into the lot. Once parked, you'll often find others standing around waiting for a minivan that will magically show up every few minutes to transport new people to the set. It's a nice little system that keeps the actual set free of unwanted vehicles. Also, transportation captains and drivers are some of the coolest and most knowledgeable people you'll meet.

If you are a principal actor, the night before your work date you would have received a call from one of the assistant directors giving you your call time for the work day. They'll usually fax you a map to the set if you're shooting somewhere on location. Jot down their name. Background players will have heard from the extras casting coordinator for the shoot.

Assistant directors, or ADs as they're better known, are almost always your first and last contact on-set. They are paid to expertly handle all the stuff that the director doesn't have time to do. The lion's share of their work is keeping track of the actors—from extras to stars. If you're cast as an extra, you'll probably be dealing with the second or second second AD. If you're playing a principal role, it will be the first AD on-set and one of the seconds for checking in and out. Like everything else, this can change with each set, but more often than not this is the accepted set structure. There are also key production assistants who sometimes are given control of extras. By keeping your eyes and ears open, you'll find out quickly enough who does what on each individual set. It's remarkable how similar this process works from shoot to shoot and set to set.

Actors with speaking roles will find nice accommodations, usually a semiprivate trailer (small individual rooms, sometimes separated by dividers) and occasionally a private trailer, a room, or a partitioned-off holding area. On most occasions, a contract and all other paperwork will be in your trailer. Fill out these papers when you have time and have your identification (driver's license, social security card, or passport) available to show the AD. Most will take it and make a copy in the production trailer, but sometimes they'll just give it a quick glance.

Background players are often held in some large room and then brought closer to the set when shooting commences. They may use the entire group at once or just a few at a time. Only in the rarest of occasions are background performers and principals sharing the same waiting area.

Let's assume you've landed an extra role on one of your favorite television series. All the stars are milling about, right there in front of you. Remember, you're now a coworker not a fan, so act accordingly. It's important to remember these folks get approached all the time. They're probably busy and don't need the distractions of being followed around by an autograph seeker. It's fine to say hello or maybe even acknowledge their fine work, but don't overstay your welcome and know when to make a graceful exit. On rare occasions, a star may strike up a conversation with you and want you to chat for awhile. That's a different story, but it's important that you recognize the difference. There are lines of demarcation that, although not always fair, are very real. A dayplayer will generally have more flexibility on a set than an extra, and a guest star will have more than a costar. You'll quickly learn what's acceptable and what isn't as you work your way up through the ranks. Stars can pretty much do anything they'd like, but then again they bring the people into the theatre at the Cineplex.

There is an unwritten doctrine on sets that must be addressed. Background performers, whether right or wrong, should not bother the director at any time. The second assistant directors are there to deal with all background performer requests. Directors don't hate extras; they just don't have the time to deal with them. There are exceptions to every rule, however, and once again it deals with the "first approach" situation. If the director comes up to you and begins talking, don't freeze and look for help. Enjoy your opportunity and spend as much time with him as is comfortable.

Principal players, however, have the ear of the director, but only to a degree. Each performer must figure out how much and when to approach the top man. A dayplayer must know when to speak up and when to defer to a guest star actor who is after the director. So, too, must a guest star back away when one of the show's film's stars wants quality director time. It's like a little kingdom in there. It's not confusing; it's common sense. On-set, you should be aware that the director's priorities first lie with his regular cast and then with the other players. A good director will make some time for all his principal players, but if you have an unanswered pertinent question and it looks like he's not going to address you, then by all means speak up before the cameras burn any film.

Actors who are brought in for background work on television series can benefit from the regular extras—those actors who have become daily workers on the shows in nonspeaking roles. These performers know the sets better than anyone, having sometimes worked multi-year contracts. They are treated nearly as well as the stars, know all the personnel, and usually have those great show jackets, too. Regular extras (when approached pleasantly) will let new people know which set phones are okay to use, what craft services are safe to graze, and sometimes they'll even tip you as to what you need to do to get called back again.

Whether you're a principal waiting in a trailer or an extra sitting in a holding area, you don't have to stay in one place all day without moving. Just stay within earshot and eyesight of the ADs. There will be times during the day when you'll need a break, a trip to the bathroom, or just a chance to stretch your legs. Just tell someone in charge that you're stepping away for a moment to take care of business. Do not disappear for half an hour just because you were told that they won't be needing you for awhile. Murphy's law always applies on film sets. You might be sitting around for five hours doing nothing, but if you sneak off without alerting someone, that's exactly when they'll be looking for you. Nothing will get you in hot water faster or, if you're an extra, maybe tossed off the set. Also, remember to never move around when the red shooting light is on. Boom mikes can pick up the subtlest of noise from a very long distance. On location, where there's no red light, stop in your tracks when you hear "Rolling."

After rehearsals, principal performers will usually be excused for awhile. It could be for half an hour while they light or for several hours if the scene isn't going to be shot for awhile. That doesn't mean that you should leave the location. You are there for the day, even if you won't be filming until the tenth hour. On rare, rare occasions, if they are absolutely sure you won't be needed for many hours, an AD may grant a request for a principal actor to leave location and return later. If you request this, it had better be for important business. Even so, they often can't let you go because the director could change his mind about the shooting order at any moment. Background performers will never leave the location until they have finished for the day and have been signed out.

Generally, when you are finished the rehearsal, they'll try to give you a ballpark on how long it's going to be. But with all the things that happen on a film set, it could much longer. It's never shorter. Find a place to relax or study your lines, but above all conserve your energy. You're going to want it when your scene comes up. Again, if you are going to be anywhere other than in your trailer, let someone know.

I'm talking a lot about being ready to go and reachable when they need you. That's very important because waiting around is such a big part of the work day. This isn't theatre where you come in and do it. In television and film, they call actors in very early to get them ready to work, but the time to actually perform will seem like forever on some shoots. The phrase "hurry up and wait" is very applicable and one you'll hear on many sets. They'll rush you into makeup and hair, get you into wardrobe, and then you'll sit waiting for an eternity. The crew members never stop working throughout the long day, but the actors must bide their time until they are called.

Even while you're waiting your turn to act, you can learn a lot about the set from just watching what's going on around you. Each set has its own personality, and part of that personality is made up of the top creative team, regular cast members, and crew. Some are outgoing, talkative, friendly, and open. Others have none of those qualities, or maybe they're just tired from one of those infamous sixteen-hour work days that are so common in the business. This is where that common sense kicks in. Listen and watch the people. Some will be approachable, some will not—all will be busy to super busy at various parts of the day. A nice "good morning" will be appreciated by almost everyone, but otherwise let them do their work. Over the course of the day, you'll have a couple of chats and figure out who is easier to deal with and who is better to avoid. Each set has a nice guy, a jerk, and all types in between. Don't take anything personally. You are a temporary visitor, undoubtedly excited for the new experience of this particular set. Those people show up day in and day out, and are dealing with politics, broken cameras, not enough time, and lunch being later than it was supposed to be. Respect the different perspective and use your head. On most sets, it all flows very nicely.

A good rule of thumb is that the crafts services people, the ones who put out all those great snacks during the day, are almost always superfriendly. There is definitely a connection between food and good cheer. The food area is always easy to find—look for a crowd of people. Be alert, although most sets have tables full of food and drink for everyone on set, don't be surprised if you find some areas that have signs reading "For crew only." If there's any question in your mind, just ask the crafts service person if the food is for the performers, too. Foodstuffs usually include chips, doughnuts, bagels, nuts, candies, and all types of high-calorie, cholesterol-busting goodies as well as fruit and healthier alternatives. Stay away from the M&Ms early in the morning and don't let the great smell of coffee take you beyond what you would drink on a normal day. Most sets will allow you to take food back to your holding area or trailer. Don't leave a mess, however. People have had sandbags dropped on them for less. Let the crafts services person know how much you like and appreciate the eats—they have egos, too, just like everyone else on a film set. Don't stretch the truth though. If the food is bad, keep your mouth shut as you don't want to encourage them any further.

Actors so closely equate food with film sets because such a large portion of the day is spent sitting around waiting for actual work. However, there are many other things to do than eat. Use this time effectively—after all, you're being paid for it. You might staple pictures and resumes together, study monologues, or do some other work-oriented activity. Of course, if you need to work on lines or just get in the right frame of mind, then by all means find your own space and luxuriate in private. There's no place like a film set to find out where other casting is happening. Most actors are more than willing to share the information—it's human nature to gossip. Downtime can be used for anything reasonable, even sleep, but you must be prepared and fully alert once you're called to the set.

Just before shooting, with the extras already in place, the principal players will be called down to the set. Their stand-ins will step out as the stars step in. This is a definite perk on many shows. Having a stand-in for filming allows you to work on other things while the shots are being lit. Television series and higher-budget films have stand-ins, but don't be surprised if you're working on a low-budget shoot and find that you are your stand-in. Like rehearsal time, never expect it, but enjoy it when the situation arises. As a principal performer, you'll shoot most of your scenes in a block and then be released. Dayplayers often have the shortest working hours. You may only have a scene or two and be out of there long before the regular cast and extras.

As the day wears on, you'll inevitably begin thinking about an expanding paycheck. After the ninth hour (one-hour grace period for a meal), overtime will kick in. Overtime brings with it a sense of invigoration for actors who earlier were starting to feel punchy. Location days, in particular, can and often do go well past twelve hours. Shows shot on lots are usually quicker and more aware of actor overtime because the suits are never far away.

As an actor, you must keep close tabs on your working hours. Never count on the busy ADs to fill out your vouchers properly. You'll want to keep track of all hours worked, make sure you've logged meal breaks, wardrobe allowances, and any penalties that could mean money in your pocket. Most important, make sure that you've signed and dated the paperwork. Never forget to include your social security number or you won't get paid. Principal players have probably had their rates negotiated by an agent and may have already filled out paperwork prior to shoot day. Don't be surprised if you still have documents to fill out when on the set.

As day goes into night, or vice versa, the acting ranks will be getting shorter and shorter as the AD wraps groups of extras and some of the principal actors. After giving them a copy of your voucher, you might want to say thank you for the job. If you're interested in coming back again, now is your chance to bring it up. Hundreds of actors pass through shows every month, so to make yourself stand out, you'll need to promote yourself, albeit in a classy fashion. ADs have been known to request specific extras repeatedly because they know they're professional and dependable.

Principal actors will usually find a few minutes after they've shot their final scene to hunker down with the director. This time should be used to discuss what's going to happen on your next shooting day or any remaining questions you may have. Most directors are so on top of things that they know when to approach each principal and share a few parting words. If yours doesn't, make the first move. If you're wrapped for good, make sure you acknowledge the helmsman. No one ever gets tired of being thanked.

Overcoming Problem Areas

You've got to be really tough if you're an actor. I'm not referring to "I'll punch your lights out" tough but the kind of tough where you willingly and regularly take an objective look at your skills, advancement, or lack thereof and at yourself.

Actors don't have full-time bosses, so it's our own job to watch for problems that might develop. We must take a discerning look at the product, ourselves, and make modifications when necessary. You'll no doubt know one or two people who will give you valuable critiques when you solicit them and sometimes even when you don't, but at the end of the day you have to do most of that work yourself.

Acting teacher Daphne Eckler Kirby offers this on the subject:

> You need to be a really good problem-solver and that means having an eye on the things that are working and advancing you forward and having the ability to see whatever kind of liability exists that may be holding you back. It might be your skill level, your agent not working for you, your level of aggressiveness or laziness. Those are some of the pitfalls.

Once you identify areas that need improvement, you must make the modification on a business, not a personal, level. Let's say you've slacked off in your marketing and your audition count has dropped precipitously as a result. Rather than bemoan your fate and continue down the same path, you must become aggressive and stop the bleeding. Mail your pictures and get back to work.

What if your agent hasn't gotten you an appointment in three months? You could sit back and take it, many actors do. Is that smart? Usually not. Given hard information, and no auditions for ninety days is pretty hard, you must do something. Make the call to your agent. If you don't see a positive change and fast, then you better get into gear and find a new rep. Too many actors identify a problem, especially the one involving their agencies, and then do nothing about it. That's two steps back and no steps forward.

But what do you do if the problem hits closer to home? What if you're the essence of the problem? It's clear that acting makes you a better actor, and if you haven't worked that muscle for awhile you must get active in class or at home with some performer friends.

Sometimes you need the job a little too much. We always want the job, but if financial needs are pressing or the pressure of not having worked in months starts to overcome you it can subtly or not so subtly affect the vibe you are giving off. Casting director Jeff Gerrard reflects, "If you need the job desperately it's going to come through. I know it's hard to say you've got to let it go when the landlord is knocking on your door for rent, but if you go in too hungry it comes through the work."

Perhaps the only solution is to admit things are tough right now. No matter how you feel, you need to convince yourself, before you step into that audition, that it's only about doing a good job as an actor on that day. The result must be secondary.

From an acting standpoint, the biggest problem that shouldn't exist is going in unprepared. Some actors do this due to sheer inexperience, but in the professional realm it more often is about not doing your homework. If you're serious about this as a vocation, you cannot function in that manner.

Caster Richard Hicks says, "Some actors do not take advantage of the opportunity they have here. They seem defensive and are winging it, and often as the observer you can take a guess but you can't really tell if it's because they suck or because they didn't prepare."

Whether it's because of a lack of talent or a lack of preparation, you'd better fix it fast or your career will be a short one.

P

Photographers

Before you try to find an agent or meet your first casting director, you will need the services of a superb photographer to shoot your headshots. After all, there are tens of thousands of pictures landing on Los Angeles casters' desks every day. You need yours to stand out from the masses.

A terrific photographer should bring three things to the table. First, he will have that magical blend of artistry and craftsmanship that will give you the absolute best picture you can achieve. Second, he will know what the market bears right now—that is, which type of headshots are being used most often and which are achieving the best results. Third, he will have top-notch equipment and studio facilities.

Top notch these days might mean digital photography. The standard is still a photographic film headshot, but the industry is quickly heading digital. Most shooters today will snap you with a film camera, others are only working digitally, and some are shifting between both mediums. Whatever format it comes out on, a great headshot is a great headshot. Don't over concern yourself with film versus digital. Focus on the photographer.

It's not difficult at all to locate a headshot photographer who'll suit your needs. The city is teeming with them. *The Working Actors Guide* and *Backstage West* are solid resources for lists of photographers' names and numbers. The better photographers are all over the Internet now. You can also find the Web site addresses in BSW and WAG, and can access the work of many photographers online to see how they stack up against one another. This is a great time saver, but you're still going to want to see actual headshots you can hold in your hand. There's no substitute for the finished product.

Your fellow actors in class and at auditions are excellent sources for seeing many different headshots. If you like one or two actors' headshots, you'll have a good chance of getting similar results from the same photographers.

I recommend that you schedule interviews with three photographers. If you absolutely love the first one you meet, you can always cancel the other two meetings. When you go into the office, you'll see a book full of headshots, photos hanging on the wall, or both. Study the evidence closely. Are the headshots full of life? Do they seem marketable? Are they in focus? You'd be surprised. You'll hear everyone from caster to director say it's about the eyes—the window to the soul. The whole picture is important, but the eyes should tell a story. They often are the thing you're drawn to in one picture over another.

Also, look to see if the photographer has only chosen one or two types of actors with whom to work. Some are better at working with certain types. You know your type. Do you see it there in the books or on the wall? If a photographer only has headshots of character men and you're a beautiful ingénue, this may not be the place for you. Most busy photographers usually have examples of all types of talent.

I also pay attention to wardrobe in the shots. When you're shooting, the photographer will have you change clothing a few times to achieve different looks. When you're interviewing, you should be looking to see if the headshots have actors in clothing that isn't too flashy, inappropriate, or boring. These days three-quarter shots are popular, and a lot of clothing is seen in the picture. So don't ignore that aspect. Yes, it's about your face, but there are other things in that picture.

Look at the makeup, too, especially on the women, as men often only use a bit of base, if anything. In my opinion, makeup shouldn't be noticeable in the pictures you are studying. Good makeup enhances, it doesn't draw attention to itself. These are acting headshots after all, not high-fashion layouts.

The bottom line to choosing will be a combination of all those factors and one other—the pictures you're seeing should excite you. They should draw you in and make the idea of going anywhere else seem anticlimactic. The photographer might be the greatest person in the world and you may hit it off like old friends, but the pictures are the final test. Remember, he's showing you what he feels are his absolute best work. What do you think?

In the end, I ask myself this: "If I were an agent, would I consider bringing this actor in solely by the photo?" That usually helps me make the choice.

The beauty of finding a great headshot is that the proof is right there in front of you. When you find someone's work that you really admire, you determine the price, and if it's affordable, schedule the shoot for a later date. Prices are across the board. There are celebrity shooters who charge into the thousands, but you needn't go that route, although you'd be guaranteed a nearly perfect result. I've never had that kind of budget for headshots but have always managed to get superb work done for less than $500. You can spend well less than that, too. Most top shooters charge in the $250–$400 range. Some are even less than that, especially someone who is trying to build up their business in a very competitive field of its own.

Get to know the photographer's personality at this meeting as well. A good shooter should spark you a bit because he or she will need to do that in the actual session. If the person doesn't inspire you in some way (funny, bright, passionate, or whatever), you may have four rolls of shots that are technically wonderful but lacking that something extra that seem to come when you're working with a photographer who can keep you fired up during the shoot. It usually comes down to a comfort level with the person. If they make you feel loose, you are going to have a fun and productive shoot.

Before you hire the photographer, there are some questions you should ask:

- *How many rolls is he going to shoot?* Two or three is a good bet. They'll do more if you request it, but a solid shooter should be able to get many excellent pictures from a three-roll outing. They'll always shoot more if you'd like, but the price will also increase. If they're shooting digital there's no film involved, so you'll be using time instead of rolls as a gauge. Shooting digitally means more pictures being taken, which that in turn means more selections from which to choose. Nevertheless, with photography it's quality not quantity that matters.

- *What is the full price, and what does it include?* You don't want any late-in-the-game surprises on pricing. Get the full price in writing and a clear description of everything that's yours. You'll need to know how many actual retouched headshots you'll walk out the door with. Many include at least two headshots in the package price. You can get more, but the price will go up.

- *Does the price include touch-ups, makeup, and hair?* In fact, does he do the retouching? Retouching is not making you look different. It's clearing up slight imperfections in the image. If the shooter doesn't do retouching, you may have to take the pictures elsewhere to get it done. Some photographers have a makeup and/or hair person on-call; if so, it usually means more expense. You can consider doing it yourself or, in some rare cases, the photographer will do the makeup for you.

- *It's important for you to be clear as to who gets the negatives (many actors like to retain the negatives for future use).* Some shooters try to keep them, but most are glad to get rid of them. Ask. You'll always want to get the negatives, even if there is an additional charge. However, once you have a retouched 8 × 10 in your possession, a printer can easily scan it, thereby leaving no need for that particular negative. You'll still want the negs though so that you can print any other proof sheet shots you didn't need this time around but might want to use in the future. You'll also want to make sure to leave with your proof sheets, but this should never be an issue. The last point will be moot if the photographer is shooting digital instead of film. In that case, there will be no negative and you'll be given a CD-rom to take to the printer.

- *Will you be shooting in the studio or outdoors?* I had one photographer who insisted on shooting everything outdoors in a park he was fond of. He was good, but that wouldn't work for me. A combination of both is nice if time permits.

- *Is there a guarantee of a free reshoot if you aren't happy with the results?* All legitimate photographers will give a reshoot without question if there were any technical problems. Some are more hesitant to do so if it's because the actor thinks her shots just aren't good. Find out and get it in writing.

All these issues are commonly addressed by the photographer, but keep these questions in mind in case he doesn't broach all the subjects to your satisfaction. If he doesn't broach any of them, go elsewhere.

To do his job most effectively, a photographer will try to get to know you a bit. Elliot de Picciotto, a Los Angeles photographer, better known as "Elliott the Retoucher," explains the partnership involved in getting to great results:

> A photographer who specializes in shooting actors should understand or at least make an effort to understand where the actor is coming from—their career goals, personality, etc. He should also be asking questions about the types of roles you feel best suited for and the types of roles you think you'd like to go for.

If the photographer insists that you pay the entire fee upfront, and many do, make sure that free reshoot guarantee is in writing, because you probably will not get your money back if things don't work out. But things work out much more often than they don't, and actors often become loyal customers for years. The competition among photographers for their share of the headshot market means good work is the norm. With due diligence and common sense, you'll find your perfect photographer from many worthy candidates.

Pilot Season

Pilot season generally falls between January and April. The networks have tons of newly conceived television projects they cast and shoot during this time frame. Most never make it to a television screen the next fall, but that doesn't matter because it's potential work for you. All it takes is one picked-up pilot and you might find yourself as a regular cast member on a real show. Normally, blasé veteran actors even get a little bounce in their step when the pilot Breakdowns start coming in shortly after the holiday season.

But let's be frank about pilot season. Although it's undoubtedly one of the busiest times of the casting year, the increase in activity often applies only to a handful of actors. If you're twenty and you look like a cross between Liv Tyler and Heather Graham, you're going to do very well during pilot season. If you're a very talented tyke, you'll likely see a lot of activity as well. If you are on the very short list of actors who get brought in repeatedly, pilot season is always a welcome time. For everyone else, it's pretty much business as usual.

Casting director Brian Myers offers some perspective on pilot season:

> There are absolutely the same actors over and over again being seen for pilots, but I think it's also a time of year when people who aren't necessarily viewed as series regular material can get seen. Because later down the line if a producer says, "Well why didn't we see that person?"—you don't want to hear that. Some producers don't want to see a lot pf people. So then unfortunately you will only be seeing actors from bigger agencies, people that are proven—that's the pool that gets dipped into every year.

If you're like most—the average actor—you might get a few more hits than normal. If you're an inexperienced newcomer to Los Angeles, hoping to break in while they're busy casting the new pilots for the upcoming television season, you might not get a single audition or meeting. But get a little excited because hope springs eternal, after all.

The sensible approach to pilot season is to be prepared for it just in case a great opportunity presents itself. This means being in class and appearing in a theatrical production during the early months of the year so that you are already working. When you're already working on your craft, you subconsciously let go a little more and don't need the job quite as much. You're also a better actor for it. Other performers come off of December, which is a very slow month, and wait for their first pilot audition to kick them back into gear. Auditions are not the place to get up to speed; you have to already be there.

I also think a mailing to casting directors during early January is a smart move. It's a chance to remind some people who may have forgotten you, or perhaps have yet to meet you, of your existence. If you're in a play, this is an even better way to promote yourself. Using a new photograph during pilot season, that shows you with a slightly different look, can be a way to get some directors to bring you in for roles for which they might not previously have thought were your type.

The mailing is good not only for pilot season, but also because this is when the current season's shows are into their second half of filming. Even if you don't get a pilot shot, you may get a caster to bring you in for a currently running program.

During pilot season, many actors from around the country buy into the hype and rush to LA to try to land an audition. The Oakwood Apartments, a famous complex for short-term visitors, swells with kids and their parents. The kids might have a shot because so many youngsters are read, but it's only those who have gotten an agent's interest. No one, child or adult, has any chance out here without a representative during pilot time. Never come here in the first quarter of the year and expect to meet agents or managers. They are swamped trying to get their existing clients auditions. If they're not swamped, you probably don't want to be signed with them anyway. Adult actors would be better served coming to LA almost any other time of the year and staying. Short stays always result in disappointment, but it's even harsher when the expectations are inflated as they tend to be during pilots.

Producers

Producers are pretty cool people, as long as you're doing your job. On a set of frenzied activity, where the bottom line is never far from their minds, producers seem to be the coolest cats on the set. They must account and answer for everything that is happening to the higher-ups, yet they manage to remain calm and collected. The good ones can control their world with a knowing glance and the flip of their Startac.

Sometimes, they show their set strength, they blow, and the heads roll. But more often when things are amiss, they usually get the ugly stuff done in a discreet fashion. A crew member or actor might be gone with nary a notice. But for all the money spent on these Hollywood productions, heads don't roll as often as you'd think. A good producer hires good people and keeps his train moving.

Look at the credit lists of any film or television show and you can become exhausted with the number of producers. There are executive producers, producers, associate producers, supervising producers, line producers, co-producers, and so on. You do not need to drive yourself crazy trying to figure out which is which. One will certainly be more noticeable, and that's the producer with whom you'll possibly deal.

Generally speaking, the executive producer, whether he is independent or an employee himself, oversees the producer who oversees the set—creatively, financially, administratively, and otherwise. The producer is also responsible for all the other producers that work under him.

During television callbacks, you'll inevitably meet the producers who in most cases are also the writers or show creators, and they'll usually make the casting decisions. Television is called a producer's medium for good reason. They call the shots. In feature films, you may not see a producer until you arrive on-set and, depending on how powerful the director is and how he likes to run his set, producers may not be very visible.

As an actor, you may go through years of your career without ever having had a real conversation with an on-set producer. They are always around there watching, but the chance of a guest actor having a face-to-face, sit-down chat with one is slight. That changes immediately when you become a series regular or star.

The producer may be sitting in his chair, often chatting with the director about shots, budgets, locations, and trailers and dealing with various department heads simultaneously, and he'll very possibly acknowledge you, but he'll generally be too busy to deal with you. As the average actor on-set, you probably won't need to be dealt with anyway. You've heard that no news is good news. It's true.

You'll make a fan of a producer if you're doing your job well and not making your presence something that he has to deal with. You're the director's charge for the day, and the producer simply won't have to worry about you, as long as you do your job. If you don't, or if you're one of those actors who just causes trouble, you may find yourself face to face with the producer for the wrong reasons. Stars might be able to get away with throwing their weight around, but a working-class actor in Hollywood is there to act and not make waves.

There are exceptions, times when you need to be an on-set businessman before you're an on-set actor. After all, this is your livelihood. Most of the business stuff is taken care of well before you step onto a set. Your agent and manager should see to that. However, sometimes things happen on the set that need your immediate attention. You may not be able to reach your agent on the phone, nor will it always be practical. In this case, you might need to speak to the producer. If there is a problem with your contract, you're asked to do something like a stunt, or there's something with which you're not comfortable, you owe it to yourself to speak up. Some actors, especially newer ones, are understandably a little intimidated about this prospect, but you have to be adult and remember that your career is more important than this one day on a set. Naturally, you want to be a team player and to not be disruptive, but I'll tell you this, everyone from the art director to the grips to the caterer to the director himself speaks up on their behalf when things aren't kosher, why shouldn't you? That doesn't mean you rush up to a producer and start complaining. This would be foolish. Creative issues would usually be brought to the director's attention, whereas business issues would be brought to the assistant director. Although the AD can usually resolve it, if he cannot, he will present it to the producer who will address the issue with you. If you don't get a resolution, particularly if it's something that presents danger, such as a stunt, go directly to the producer before you proceed.

Public Transportation

Public transportation, long derided and ridiculed in Los Angeles, isn't nearly as bad as people say. This doesn't mean you'll want to use it as an actor. Sandra Bullock did in *Speed* and you saw what happened to her!

As a surviving performer, you can't rely on public transport. You, like most others, will own or lease an automobile, a motorcycle, a Vespa, or anything that you can steer. If you think for a minute you can get by without your own mode of transportation in show business you are sadly mistaken. You must have something nearby to carry you to last-minute auditions and work calls. You can theoretically get anywhere in the city using public transportation, but it could take you hours. It's impossible to structure a career around that restriction.

LA has a vastly improved bus and train system and the slickest-looking subway in America, but none of those are practical for the acting life. Use them when you have time to explore the city of Los Angeles, but until there is a subway stop on every corner, taking you to all points in the city, hold onto your driver's license.

I didn't tell you this, but when you see one of those new red express buses that are appearing, especially on Wilshire Boulevard, you might want to follow a safe distance behind them. They do not have a little driver device that can keep green lights from turning red.

Q

Quiet Acting

They always say the best actors are the ones that can listen, and there's a lot of truth to that. But eventually you'll have to speak. When it's your turn in front of the camera for the first time, it's important to remember the wonderful world of amplification. You have been miked. As such, you needn't project the way you would for a stage performance. In fact, in most cases, you can have a very normal level of conversation even when you think you should be projecting a bit because you are performing after all. You could project as sometimes volume is even encouraged (shoot 'em up scenes or around noisy machinery, or maybe you're just supposed to be yelling at someone), but a lot of what you'll be doing will be plain old normal-level speech. Sooner or later, a friendly director will remind you of that.

Quiet acting also applies to the casting process. There are two kinds of rooms casting directors use—very small and very big. The big rooms might lead you to speak more loudly, but remember that you're reading for the camera not the stage. You don't want to come off like Master Thespian! The small spaces cause you to speak more quietly. Maybe that's intentional on the casters part or maybe their bosses won't spring for a roomier office. Who knows? Whatever the case, don't make it so your voice is so low that people need to lean forward to hear you.

Quick Results

The average actor usually gets only a modicum of rehearsal and maybe a few attempts to get the job done. You've got to be a quick study and an adaptable actor to be successful in Hollywood. If you learn to deliver the goods quickly, cleanly, and consistently, this will make everyone very happy, most of all you.

You have to go from inactivity to being up to full speed at a moment's notice and, on top of that, you're acting and you must excel at it. The evidence of your efforts might live on in syndication and cable for the rest of your life. With the sun rising over the horizon there is no room for error or retakes. They are paying you to be a pro and nail it the first time. If you can do that and do it consistently, you'll work in Hollywood. You need to be able to work fast, work well, and do your part to keep the project on budget and on schedule. Surviving actors either have the knack for getting quick results or they learn it real fast when the skillet hits the flame.

One particularly fast-paced environment where the mettle of any actor would be tested is the live variety show. One-hour episodes are fast and sitcoms are faster, but a live variety show is the fastest and it's live.

A perfect example of this is NBC's "The Tonight Show with Jay Leno," for which Talent Coordinator Scott Atwell casts hundreds of actors per year, primarily for the short sketches that have become a hallmark of the program. The casting is fast and the work happens at breakneck speed. Performers need to be sharp and reliable if they are going to succeed. As Atwell says,

> We're so fast paced here. We tape year round and it's a constant. We cast anywhere from twenty five to seventy five under-five actors a week. I can go though five pictures for the same role in ten minutes if I'm not getting an answer from a telephone call. Performance wise, the people who thrive here are just really strong actors. They're also really funny and are able to click with the writers or whoever is directing the piece. An improv and comedic background is always a plus.

The improvisation Atwell refers to can carry an actor through a lot of tough spots during a career, especially when the clock is ticking and you need to deliver the goods fast. With improvisation, you are ready for almost anything. Even if you're heading down the wrong performance track, your training will often quickly guide you back to a solution.

Quotes

Quotes are the pay rate an actor earns for his employment on a film or television show. Theoretically, the more you work, the higher you should be paid, and the higher your quote goes. Until the 1990s, that's just the way it worked for many years until Hollywood studios started tightening their economic belts when it came to costars and guests stars.

The studios claim it's harder and harder to make a buck these days. Yeah, tell us about it. The two most common excuses for this phenomenon, which the industry sweetly refers to as "salary compression," are the escalating costs of production and the fact the megastars are eating up the talent budget with their $20 million paychecks. I think I believe about half of each of those excuses. Production costs are growing out of control and stars do receive a huge amount of the funds, but incredible profits can still be realized from hit television and film sales in the United States and abroad. If the stars cut their fees in half, that money wouldn't likely be filtered back into the rest of the acting community.

The bottom line is that today it's harder and harder for agents to get their noncelebrity clients their quotes. Consequently, the average actor must choose between taking less money for the job than he has gotten in the past or turning down the work altogether. Not many surviving actors can afford to turn down work, and producers know this.

In case you think the quotes I'm referring to are thousands of dollars per day, you'd be wrong. Generally, it's in the hundreds or just creeping up into the four-digit range for most average actors. Even actors that a few years ago were making substantially more are now resigned in some instances to having to make a living off of union scale—that's as little as they can legally pay a member of SAG or AFTRA.

It's a real challenge for the average actor and agents who do all they can to press producers to pay the appropriate quotes. Agents are often forced to present an offer to their clients that is no reflection on the dues they have paid.

As agent Kurt Patino aptly points out,

> There's not enough green to go around, so they stick it to the day player. "That kind of money was not budgeted for this role," casting directors will say. It's simple negotiation. If the deal's not good enough, you walk away, and then hope that they want you enough to give you what you're worth. Sometimes, you just have to call their bluff. Other times, it might be the experience or the quality that you're really after in a project. It's up to you.

In a business where unemployment is the norm, there are times when a noncelebrity actor would have to be glad to hear them say *all* they're offering is scale plus ten percent because that would mean they want to hire you. Perhaps after a long break from work, some actors will jump at any offer, even scale, but they have to be careful how often they jump. If you continually support working for less than your quote rate, then others will, too, and the result of that could be the elimination of quotes for all but the major players. Some think we're headed in the direction of scale for all but the stars. That might seem kind of far-fetched even today, but things can change if people stop paying attention. So before you take a no-quote job (that's where they don't keep a record of what they paid you for others to confirm), consider how badly you need the work and whether you can afford to turn it down. You are a professional after all.

Like any other profession, the longer you do this, the better you get, and the more you should be compensated for your work. This does happen, thanks to the producers who can afford to or choose to do the right thing. There are some that don't balk at paying the actor their quote rate and maybe even a bit more to show they respect and follow the quotes system. This isn't about a low-budget producer asking for a pay break on talent for a microbudgeted show. Almost any actor would jump in and work for less than their quote on a quality project that has verifiably slim production and talent funds. However, when a multimillion-dollar network program cries poor mouth to an agent saying they can't pay $800 for a professional actor's services, it's kind of hard to believe. Especially when they're giving some civilian $2000 to shoot in their front yard and filming it from a rented helicopter.

An actor may not be employed again for a week, a month, or a year. That's why getting your rightful quote is so important. It's survival.

R

Rejection

Surviving actors get rejected on an almost daily basis. People smile at you, tell you what a fine job you did, and then don't hire you. It happens to us all the time, and yet we come back bouncing and ready for the next go round.

Actors face rejection with aplomb, class, and a sense of humor. Humans don't always fare so well, and I'm guessing you're human as well as an actor.

Being rejected stinks. Even if you know it's a professional rejection not a personal one. But here's the rub. It's a normal part of being an actor in Hollywood. Until you reach that ultrastar level of acting, you will be turned down far more than you will be accepted. The average actor in television would be considered successful by hiring standards if he got only one-tenth of the jobs he auditioned for, one-fiftieth or even more if he was vying for work in commercials. So know going in that you will be said "no" to a lot more than you will ever be given a W2 form to fill out.

Rejection though, in whatever form, can start to work on you. You've always got to stay strong and prove it on a daily basis by facing the rejection head on.

As you gain more experience in the field, you'll learn to better deal with being rejected. It rolls off a little easier. You'll always want to book the job, but you'll begin to grasp that it's not so much about the result but about the effort you made. If you do your best job as a prepared actor in the audition and still don't get the job, just chalk it up to the statistical norm. You'll still know you gave a good day at the office. When you start to do this, you'll become a more total package actor.

Residuals

While writing this book, I had the occasion to speak with a British actor whom I met when filming a television series. In our conversation, I asked him how the acting market was in the United Kingdom. Could one make a decent living there? He didn't miss a beat before telling me that there is certainly work, but as far as making a living, well, he'd come to Hollywood to do that. It turns out that in Britain there is no residual system at all. The actor makes what he makes when shooting a project and then never sees another dollar.

That would send a shudder through any American actor. For all the respect accorded all performing artists throughout much of Europe, respect alone doesn't pay the bills.

In the United States, where a reported ninety-five percent of union members make less than $5000 per year, it is virtually impossible to make a monetary living without residual payments. Nonunion actors do not get residuals, which is yet one more reason so many are clamoring to join.

Residuals are a crucial necessity for the surviving actor. A few super-stars might get their $25 million per film and a nice percentage of the first dollar box office gross, but almost all other performers make what they make from their shoot day session fees (often scale or maybe the actor's current quote) and then rely heavily on residuals to pay their rent and bills throughout the rest of the year.

These are the lucky actors, because to get a residual means you've seen actual employment in your profession. Many don't. You'll need a lot of employment to have any chance of having those residuals amount to decent figures. The sticky wicket with residuals is that they continually shrink over the months and years. Your performances are on television throughout the years for people to enjoy, but your fiscal reward for it continually dwindles from decent, to minimal, to practically laughable. If you don't continually generate new jobs throughout your career, you might be facing residual checks in the pennies instead of dollars. There's actually a bar in the San Fernando Valley called Residuals, where actors bring in their tiniest paychecks to be hung over the bar for all to see. Cashing a check for a dime is too humiliating, so up on the wall it goes! We have a twisted sense of humor about these things.

Here are some residuals you might find in your mailbox through the years:

- *Television*—Here's a possible residual *best-case* scenario. An actor works on a successful network drama and is paid $800 for a day's work. The show might yield a payment schedule like this through the years—one network rerun (paid at the rate of one hundred percent of the original fee) and then on to syndication where payments run on a sliding scale from fifty percent to five percent as the episode runs repeatedly. Between network and syndication, an actor can do okay, but soon enough the show flops over to cable and the checks arrive annually instead of every few months. They are often so small, you'll think there was a clerical error. Looking at this one show, the actor could make perhaps a few thousand dollars after several years. Not bad, but that money is spread out over time losing its current-day value. This was a hit show—maybe as good as it gets for television show residuals. Most programs you'll work on won't have a run like that. You may end up with just one network rerun before the show goes away for good. Only the big hits get bought into syndication where that decent residual cycle can be had, for awhile anyway. Nowadays, even that's being threatened.

What's happening today, much to the consternation of working actors, is that some producers are skipping the syndication market altogether and selling directly to cable from network. The producer doesn't make as much per sale, but he also doesn't have to pay out nearly as much to the talent. This is all the more reason to get as much as you can for your quote rate when you book the job.

There are other television *surprise* residual fees that might arrive as the months and years pass. Foreign sales are one area from which an actor can expect a couple of dollars from a successful show.

- *Feature Films*—If you've worked on a film, you won't get residuals for quite awhile, at least until it leaves the theatre and moves into other areas, most notably television and video. The best thing that can happen is that the film has a long theatrical run, becomes a big hit, and is sold to the television market. When a film hits television, you can expect to get a very good residual check, especially if it airs primetime on a network. If the film bombs at the box office, an actor still might receive a small pay channel check somewhere down the line and perhaps something from the foreign market. If it was a hit, he'll also get those residuals eventually. When a film does well, everyone wins. They don't all do well, but sooner or later they all end up on the Blockbuster shelves (video and DVD), and you can expect to get a residual payment for both sales and rentals of the film. These are based on sales numbers, so if the film tanked at the box office it may also tank here. To be safe, don't count your residual until it's hatched.

- *Commercials*—The biggest residuals payments are easily found in that wonderful world of commercials. A system of airing that rates markets and runs, which is Byzantine to even the sharpest accountant, ultimately means that a long-running television or radio ad will certainly mean good bucks for the talent involved; often, much more than an actor could ever expect from a film or television residual. With commercials, they could be coming in weeks, not months or years, later. It's understandable why actors put up with massive cattle calls and callback upon callback just to land one decent commercial. The magic word for commercial residuals is *national.* If you have a spot that is airing in all or nearly all the major markets across the United States, you are going to be receiving repeated residuals. Of course, there's a flip side. Today they shoot many more commercials, but air fewer of them overall. As such, it's increasingly difficult to get a big commercial that will generate substantial residuals. Most actors are content just booking a commercial and maybe getting a regional run or wild spots.

Reviews

A surviving actor must remain thick-skinned when it comes to reviews. As a professional, particularly one who plays on stage, you'll get reviewed from time to time. If you're like most, you'll have some good notices along the way. You'll praise those reviewers for their good taste and obvious intellect.

Then when you least expect it, maybe even when you feel you're doing your best work, someone will slam you with a bad one. You'll cuss the very mention of the word critic, and you'll swear you'll never read another review again.

You may have done your best work that night, or perhaps you really did have a bad night. There may even be validity to the review, or it may be completely off base. The bottom line is that it doesn't really matter.

It was one person's opinion of work you did on a particular night. Being a writer who knows many reviewers, I'm going to take their side for a moment. Most of the time these people are very good at what they do. They're knowledgeable about the craft and the history of theatre and can objectively evaluate very well. Sometimes they're way off base or they just might have had a bad day. Again, none of it really matters. You did your performance and grew as actors do from each show they are in. What you got from it had nothing to do with a review—whether good or bad.

Of course, with reviews, other people read those words. In the case of film and television critics, others watch them on the tube, not the least of whom are the actors being reviewed. When you hear your name associated with something identified as less than wonderful, you are going to take it personally. It's understandable but you need to get past it and fast.

It really doesn't matter in the big picture, because your work stands on its own. Maybe you can even learn a thing or two from a well-written review, whether it is positive or negative. Whatever your review says, don't take them too seriously. If you let the great ones inflate you, then you'll get knocked down all that much harder when someone takes a hard punch at your performance.

I've also learned a little survival trick with reviews, aside from taking them with a grain of salt. I don't look at them until after the show closes, if at all. The work is already done, and the review won't give you any unnecessary baggage if you're staring at a four-month run and are only in the second week of the show. Of course, if the show is a huge hit, several cast members are going to arrive with copies of the review early on, so make your choice and live with it.

Runaway and Disappearing Productions

As an actor, you'll be concerned with having a great teacher, getting auditions, and staying in touch with your agent—all important things to be concerned about. There are a couple of other things of which you should also be aware. Otherwise, you might not have that other stuff to concern yourself with someday. They're called *disappearing* and *runaway productions* and they're truly threatening our industry and our livelihood.

Remember MOWs, the Movies of the Week? They were shot here in Los Angeles and throughout America, and were a staple of the surviving actor's workload. Where have they gone? Well, there are still a few left, now primarily produced by cable networks, instead of the Big Three, but they are usually lensed in Canada and overseas. When television movies were much more prolific, they were fond of casting unknown and noncelebrity actors in pivotal roles. Then they all but disappeared, almost overnight. So did a large amount of the earnings on which middle-class actors could count.

So the handful remaining were undoubtedly helped to their demise by something called unscripted reality television. You know the shows—six singles on a boat trying to score, fourteen yuppies battling in the desert, and a wealthy bachelor meeting his would-be bride via a televised catfight. This form of extremely low-cost produced *entertainment* appealed to the new corporate powers who are increasingly taking control of the film and television business. Not surprisingly, these shows are also very profitable.

At the same time as the *Survivors, Fear Factors,* and *Big Brothers* have been spreading, an increasing number of scripted television series, which kept a lot of average U.S. actors sporadically employed, began calling Vancouver, Toronto, and Sydney home. Apparently, everything from the cast and crew costs to the price of the light gels and walkie-talkies are cheaper elsewhere. Add in, or rather subtract out, tax breaks and is it any surprise they've looked abroad to film?

Most of these shows are owned by American companies and produced by people who live right here in Los Angeles, yet they take their product beyond our shores and North and South of the border. Feature films are following suit. They'll bring the director, the producers, and maybe three or four stars with them; the rest are hired abroad.

More and more domestic acting jobs are being lost, and this is in a field where, in the best of times, it's been very hard to get a gig.

It's not just actors being affected either. They are just the tip of the iceberg. Writers, gaffers, set designers, grips, camera operators, craft services people, makeup artists, and so on are also being hurt. Bottom line: thousands of professionals in our field who had work years ago, suddenly don't. This cannot be ignored.

We all have to do our part to save our shrinking industry.

Influence any industry power brokers and politicians you can to fight for domestic tax breaks that will encourage producers to shoot and keep their *scripted* projects here in the United States. By doing so, you'll be helping out our economy and our business, and possibly even generating some future work for yourself and your fellow actors in the process. Oh, and those reality shows, which don't employ actors, don't watch them.

That's my political statement for the book.

S

Safety

Part of surviving is keeping yourself alive. Film sets can be dangerous places, and actors are sometimes placed in positions where they can come into harm. When you're young or new to the business, you may ignore this stuff and always believe that there are professionals in charge who will assure your well-being. Then you'll find out that this isn't always the case.

Ask any actor you meet in Hollywood to tell you about an on-set horror story, and you'll realize that there are a whole lot of misses and near misses. Most of the time it happens when an actor is expected to do something like a stunt. Usually there are stunt people, but not always. If you find yourself on a set being asked to do something that sounds, looks, or feels dangerous, then you'd better step back and start asking serious questions.

Years ago, I was working on a film set where a director insisted on having real prop airplanes buzz the cast who were all dead, having lost a battle in World War I. The planes got lower and lower as the day progressed. Eventually they got so low that we could literally feel the prop wind as the planes came over us. I lay there thinking, am I being paid enough for this? Couldn't they use dummies? Well, they were. We were the dummies for doing it! Just as I got to the point of wanting to walk, an actor next to me stood up and shouted, "This is insane." He stormed off the set while the director, making a complete ass of himself, screamed into the megaphone to get the guy off his set. Too late, pal, he was gone. I decided that life was something I also wanted to experience more of and followed suit right behind that smart actor. At that moment, I realized I'd never do something to risk my life for a shot.

That was an eye-opening experience and the day when I finally understood that a stunt man gets paid what he does for very good reason. It's dangerous work. It's also not part of the actor's job description.

Most work situations aren't life threatening. What if someone asks you to take a near punch, jump over a row of hedges, or wrestle with another performer? Each actor has a different comfort level and each must make his own choices. Remember that sometimes experts are around to guide you and sometimes there are people who just *act* like they're experts. It's up to you to find out who is who. Ask questions long before the camera rolls and find out the true expertise of the person answering them. If you get half-answers or blank stares, you'd better be cautious about following their lead.

Mark Vanslow is an expert. This stuntman/actor has worked on the edge on "Nash Bridges" and "VIP," and has been the stunt coordinator on "The Back Lot Murders" and the "WaterWorld Live" show, which runs everyday at Universal Studios. Vanslow offers this on actors and set safety:

> It's the actor's responsibility to be honest and know his or her own limitations. If a scene calls for an actor to run along the edge of a rooftop and that actor is eager or afraid of heights, for safety's sake the actor should ask for a stunt double. The stunt double is there to protect his/her actor and to make them look good. Remember safety first. Only you know what you are fully capable of and what your limits are. Your body is your instrument and you make your livelihood from that instrument.

On most sets, if you're in a scene that requires anything potentially dangerous, there will be a stunt double waiting for you when you arrive on-set. However, if you work long enough in the film business, you could find yourself being asked to do something that seems questionable to your health and well-being, and there won't be anyone in sight. Aside from stunts, this could apply to working around explosives, special effects, or heavy equipment with which you're not familiar.

Take a deep breath, look around, and remind them that you've been hired to act. Don't be intimidated by anyone into making a foolish decision. Make an adult choice based on smarts, not on blind trust or for nonsensical fear that you'll never work in Hollywood again. If you get seriously hurt, you may not have a chance to work again anywhere.

Self-Esteem

Deep inside you know that you're a solid person. You know you're talented, dedicated, and going to succeed because of all your hard work. But there's that little voice that creeps in every so often that says, "What are you doing? You don't really think you're going to make it do you? When's the last time anybody hired you to do this, you, you person that dares call yourself an actor?"

The truth is, of course, everyone battles with self-esteem issues once in a while, but there is no other vocation in which one's success so closely ties in with feelings of self-worth. It's because our profession goes beyond a job—it's an emotion married to a craft connected to a business.

Imagine someone in practically any other field going to the office each day only to find a big, burly guard telling them to head home because there's no need for their services. This happens daily to the professional actor. We are told, *"no,"* almost every day. Actors put their hearts on the line every time they step before a group of strangers to audition. They do more than read a part. They invest a part of their soul and they expose themselves, and more often than not they get a smile and a wave to go on their way.

You think this is not going to affect your self-esteem over the long run? It certainly does. You're not a rock, so you'd better accept it, push through it, and remember that even amidst the *"nos,"* what you do is indeed special. Aside from a few who act for all the wrong reasons, actors do what they do to move people and that's enough reason to pick yourself up again.

You're going to have bad days, days when your self-esteem is bordering on curb height. You cannot ignore it, but you also can't let it rule you. What's more, you cannot begin to allow yourself to be defined by how much work you book. That's a dangerous proposition, because like all actors, even if you're red hot, sooner or later you're going to slow down. If you're starting to let your self-esteem be controlled by other's decisions, you are in for a tough haul. Others can't do that if you don't allow them. When you are better able to detach from the result of the audition, you go a long way toward turning the table on sagging self-esteem.

Actors sometimes get a rap as being insecure and needy. To anyone who believes that, I suggest they step up the plate and try making it in this business for one month. The full-time actor will be the one who is there to prop them up when they're falling.

Sexual Harassment

In the introduction to this book, I mentioned how great the industry and city we've chosen can be. I also mentioned that it can get ugly. Sexual harassment is maybe the ugliest aspect. There are actually very smart people here who ignore the obvious, and choose to look at Hollywood through rose-colored glasses. They've actually made themselves believe that sexual harassment is a thing of the past in the acting world. How wrong can they get?

It's alive all right. Actresses and, to a lesser degree, actors must be aware of it early on to protect themselves if they ever encounter it. In an industry with a lot of beautiful people who are looking for a way to become successful, there are those who will promise them the world to satisfy their own twisted needs.

I can't tell you how many letters I've received at *Backstage West* throughout the years. I'm not talking about borderline cases here, but flagrant, blatant examples of sick people trying to use another human. Know it exists, don't let it ever befall you, and you will have a great career.

Most of the harassers are fringe people—not real players, but con artists, liars, and sometimes already convicted crooks. They'll set up a shop and seek out the most gullible newcomers. That's pretty bad. What's worse, though, are the few people who are actual legitimate professionals in show business who do the same thing. Although few in number, they exist and they'll coerce, intimidate, humiliate, and sometimes threaten to get what they want. As a surviving actor, you have to keep them out of your circle.

Sexual harassment isn't peculiar to the acting business. It exists in all industries. It exists in the entertainment corporate world, but there's a difference between those environments and the average actor's world. When sexual harassment happens elsewhere, the employees will find a formal mechanism and process for reporting the incident(s). Actresses are often on their own, and they're often scared. The reason—the fear that has always floated just above the smog line—if I say something about it I'll be blackballed. Harassers in Hollywood know that fear exists, and they exploit a lot more people because of it.

Don't fear a land shark. If you meet one and he tries anything, get him out of your life immediately. Leave his office. Don't take his phone calls. Keep him out of your life, no matter who he says he knows, represents, or can introduce you to.

If for some reason you cannot walk away, you do have recourse even though you're not an employee. There are lawyers, the City Attorney's Office, and always the police should you be threatened or physically attacked in any fashion. If there is any physical contact what-soever, which legally constitutes battery or sexual battery, you can also contact the Special Enforcement Unit of the City Attorney's Office. SAG also has a Sexual Harassment Hotline.

Sides

Sides are the audition material you'll be supplied when you land an audition. They can be anything from a single page to multiple pages from the script. In fact, sometimes you'll get access to a full script, but for smaller parts that's not common.

However you receive your audition sides, via fax (either from your agent or directly from the caster), the Internet (from one of the companies that sell sides such as Showfax and Castnet), or even by driving over to the casting director's office (does anyone do that anymore?), they'll usually be accessible at least twenty-four hours before your audition for television projects. Be aware, though, that due to the nature of television rewrites you might arrive for the actual audition and be given totally different lines.

For feature film auditions, sides are usually available several days in advance because the script has been completed well before the auditions. Rewrites also occur here on occasion, but if they do you'll usually know well in advance. Full scripts are also more accessible in the film world if you want to read it before your audition.

For almost all commercials, the average actor will see the material for the first time when he arrives for the audition.

With television and film sides, the casting director will almost always boldly mark a start and stop point on the sides. This is your scene(s), but you might want to read what happens just before and after your part, which can sometimes provide more insight into your character. Sometimes the caster will include a page or two from a scene just before or after yours that might provide critical information about your character. It doesn't happen all the time but when it does you should take advantage of this extra information.

Your sides should not be used as a placemat for lunch. They are your lifeline to work. Use them. Rehearse with them. Visit an acting coach with them, but do something with them because the other actors reading for the part certainly are. Only the prepared ones are going to have a real shot at getting a callback. Even if it's just a few lines, don't get lazy and wait to look at the sides for the first time when you arrive at the office. If it's a last second rewrite, that's one thing. When you've been supplied material beforehand, they'd like you to know it.

Because you've been given access to these valuable pieces of paper, you might also remember to bring them with you into the audition room. Some actors stick them in their pocket and to their horror forget lines halfway through the audition. The scramble to dig the sides out of a pocket and find your place isn't pretty. Do what smart actors do and keep the sides in your hand, and use them as your backup. Because you've rehearsed beforehand, you shouldn't need to read from the page too much. If you were lazy in your preparation you'll be doing a reading, *literally,* and that won't get you much further than a free parking validation.

Stars

One day you're watching your favorite movie star in a film and the next you find yourself having been hired to act opposite him. This is a time an actor never forgets—the first professional encounter with a name performer. In a blink, you've gone from fan to colleague. Buckle up, buddy, you've arrived in Los Angeles.

There are plenty of reasons to be excited about working with a big name, not the least of which is that scenes with them often survive—meaning they usually make it through the edit into the final cut. Shortly thereafter, they appear at the top of your demo reel.

None of the training, theatre experience, or previously booked on-camera work will fully prepare you for your first time with an icon. I remember one of my first. This lovely lady immediately broke the ice for me by coming up and saying, "I'm really glad you're here." I melted from the warmth and still managed to remember my lines.

Here's the good news. Stars are just actors, too, but they're a little more successful than most. Okay, they're *a lot* more successful. You cannot help but be momentarily impressed by their presence. You've enjoyed them for years and their work has moved you. It's completely natural that there will be a period when you are awed that you are actually going to do a scene with one of these people.

The survival skill is to acknowledge it and then get past it. If you can't get the grin off your face, I'm sure someone from makeup will paint it off for you. Because you are a fellow actor, you should behave as one. There will obviously be none of the autograph or "can you help me get a better agent?" stuff. Introduce yourself, let them know you admire their work, and then get to the work at hand. If they later open up the conversation to other topics such as family, sports, or the stock market, then by all means enjoy the banter and go with it. Follow their lead and you'll be fine.

Chances are you'll go through your entire career having plenty of wonderful experiences with stars and maybe once or twice hit an attitude case. In that case, you only need remember Rule 1: They are the star and you are not. I've only met two and was still able to work with them because I'm a survivor and I like to be able to pay my rent.

Here's the better news. Stars, and I generally find the bigger the name the more this applies, are wonderful people. The major ones are secure with themselves and their careers, and often give as much as they get. They treat you as an equal and often support you, too.

I was privileged to work with an actor who showed me his nurturing spirit by his actions. It was the last shot of the morning and the crew was racing to finish up before moving onto a new location. Everyone wanted to get the shot and move on. The light was changing, too, and that really gets everybody rushing around. The camera is on me and after a fairly wordy exchange, I stumble and forget one of my lines. Rather than let me drown, this star flubs his line immediately after I flub mine. Everyone laughs, and I look at him and he gives me a little knowing half-smile. He dropped that line for me. Does it get any better than that as a Hollywood actor?

Studio Lots

Being invited to pass through the fabled gates of one of Hollywood's studios to audition for a role is the dream of most actors. You've seen those images your whole life: those fabulous gates at Paramount, the water tower at Warner Brothers, that grand back lot at Universal, and then one day you find yourself being waved through by a smiling guard who actually wishes you good luck on your audition. The only way you'll improve on that day is if they actually invite you back to work.

The lots, which are found in the San Fernando Valley, in Hollywood, on the Westside, and in surrounding communities, are the hallowed ground of acting. If you're fortunate, you'll act in many locations during your career, on the streets of the city, in suburban houses, towering office buildings, or on locations pretty much anywhere locations exist, but no single place comes close to offering the excitement and history as does working on a studio lot. As far as I'm concerned, it's a wonderful and humbling feeling that never goes away.

The bigger lots are Paramount, Disney, Universal Studios, Sony, Fox, Disney, and Warner Brothers. Then there are the so-called minilots such as CBS Radford, which has never seemed mini to anyone, and Hollywood Center Studios and Valencia Studios in the Antelope Valley. Then there are the network lots like NBC in Burbank and ABC on the Eastside.

When you get called to any studio lot for an audition, you'll pretty much encounter the same type of setup—a *drive-on* (parking on site) and a guard gate, not necessarily in that order. The guard will have your name on a list if you have a scheduled appointment.

You'll either be waved through to a designated parking area or be told to park across the street in a nearby structure and then return for a walk-on pass. You'll never park near where you'll actually be auditioning, so give yourself plenty of time and plan on a hike. Lots are huge. Don't even think about taking one of those premier parking spots near the elevator that say "Reserved." They say that for a reason.

You'll probably end up on the roof of the parking structure or across the street from the lot, as is usually the case at Warner Brothers and Paramount. If you are going to Fox, you'll end up just to the right of the guard gate where they actually have valet parking! How nice is that? Of course, you'll have to walk fifteen minutes to your audition location, but that's one of the nice perks of lot auditioning—you get to experience some Hollywood history on your way. Again, arrive early, especially the first time because you'll be unfamiliar with the layout. Otherwise, you'll find yourself huffing across the lot and sweating like a track star in front of the people for whom you're reading.

Before you park, the guard will give you directions to your appointment office. It usually goes something like, "Okay you walk all the way across the lot, past the New York Street over to Sound Stage 14 where you'll follow the blue line straight past the writer's building. Make a left at the commissary and a right at Animation Building 2. Keep going and you'll see the scene shop, don't stop, go past wardrobe, around the lumber yard, make a right at the main street and then you'll find the trailers." Just to be safe, they'll usually toss you a minimap of the lot as well. Don't leave it in your car.

You'll see everything you've ever imagined about Hollywood while on the lot. Sitcom stars yakking with their agents in the commissary, precocious kid actors sitting astride directors chairs like kings of the castle, mail being delivered via bright red bicycles, extras dressed as space aliens catching a smoke between shots, wardrobe racks rolling off trucks, amazing sets being built, directors walking empty back lot streets lining up shots for the next day. It's all a rush and, in your own way, you're part of it now. Auditioning is a pretty good start to being a survivor, and the next step, the booking, will ultimately come.

Since the tragedy of September 11, studios have been operating with varying degrees of heightened security. Gone, or at least far from the foreseeable future, are the days when an actor could find his own way onto a lot to drop a picture. Security is now so tight that you'll find it nearly impossible to get onto a lot without an appointment. It might hurt your marketing, but no one can argue that safety is the first priority now.

If you do have a scheduled appointment, you may receive a thorough search of your vehicle. The guards are exceedingly helpful and friendly. You should be the same. The process can take quite awhile. Arrive very early and have your driver's license in hand to expedite the procedure.

If you must get a picture directly to someone on the lot and mailing won't do, then you can try to drop one with the guard at the gate who will sometimes take your package. Do not attempt to evade security. No one has much reason to coddle you, and you might find yourself barred from a studio if you attempt to breach security.

Survival Jobs

Unless you come to Los Angeles with very deep pockets or have a generous relative, you will need to find and keep a survival job. It's usually easier to find one than to keep one, especially when your boss finds out you're an actor and need off for a last-minute audition.

Glenn Michael Herrera, like most actors, has relied on survival jobs to cover him between gigs:

> I would say the most important thing once you get to town is to find yourself some employment, so that you never have to worry about

eating. Find yourself some way of making money. That way you're mentally and physically in a state where you can spend all your energies going out and looking for acting work. It's hard to look when you can't pay your bills and you can't eat.

His point is well taken. You came here to act, but to do that you have to have the financial and psychological freedom to pursue your career. There has to be a balance, and you might be able to find it by sticking to the fields that traditionally hire actors—restaurants, bars, temp agencies, telemarketing, hotels, and retail. In those environments, you will no doubt find many actors doing the same thing to pay the bills. You will also discover a much higher chance for flexibility of hours.

Even if your boss cannot work with you on your schedule, being around other actors in the cafe or hotel is attractive because you can often switch schedules. You cover for one actor when he gets a same-day audition and I guarantee he'll return the favor for you. You might even get a tip on an audition you weren't aware of.

My advice is to try to be honest with your employer when you apply for a job. It's easier to be frank here because so many actors have set the precedent for this situation. Tell him you're an actor and let him know that a flexible schedule is important to you. If, however, you are really pressed for a job, it's the 25th of the month, and you don't have next month's rent money, you might want to take the job and discuss the acting thing later. Sometimes, it's about survival.

If you have an actor-friendly boss, you will usually find more support when auditions and work arrive. If you have the other kind of boss, you might have to be a little more creative when you need the occasional day off.

No actor should become married to any survival job. I have a theory that every survival job has a ticking clock on it. Sooner or later, and that might be after many years, you will have say good-bye to that gig because acting will come a knocking. There will eventually be a point where an acting job will conflict with your day job. You're an actor first, remember that. There is always another survival job.

Just a few thoughts on specific survival gigs that you might look for. I can speak with some knowledge of these jobs as I've done them, as have many actors I've known:

- *Restaurant waiter, host, bartender*—You get a flexible schedule, fellow actors working alongside and trading shifts, and a free meal each shift. You can often work at night, which means no conflict with film or television auditions, and you go home with cash in your pocket each night. There's also a very good chance that your boss will also be an actor. The downside is that late hours can put bags under your eyes.

- *Retail sales*—Successful actors are natural-born salespeople, and they usually do very well in retail. On top of that, there is a ton of retail in LA and always signs in the windows seeking help—from the chic shops to the major department stores. Usually, there's flexibility in schedule (but not as much as in the restaurant/bar business) and you get nice discounts. It's a fairly sane survival job environment compared with other fields. The downside is that rude customers can suck the life out of you. Wow, did I just say that?

- *Temp work*—This is a huge support base for actors. Regardless of your specialty, clerical, marketing, advertising, front of office, accounting, sales, etc., there is surely a temp agency that'll have openings for actors. You can make your schedule weekly, sometimes daily, and if you quit the next day no one will be too upset. In fact, they'll probably hire you back as long as you do a good job. The downside is that by the time you settle in, you're usually gone.

- *Apartment managing*—There are many apartment buildings in Los Angeles that are managed by aspiring actors. Great gigs, but you live where you work and that's a factor to consider. It's markedly more attractive if you have a significant other who can be around the building when you are off on auditions and work. You'll either get a free or heavily discounted apartment and, depending on the number of units, there can be a small to large salary involved. A big plus is that you are essentially your own boss. You'll certainly have an owner or management company to report to once in awhile (like at the first of the month when rents are sent in), but if you keep the apartments leased they'll give you all the flexibility you'll need. Remember that apartments are primarily shown on weekends, so if there are vacancies you might not see too many getaway weekends to Palm Springs. If you take a job like this, and I did for awhile, I suggest a smaller building (maybe 15 to 20) apartments with a supporting maintenance staff. That should leave you plenty of maneuverability. The downside is plumbing leaks at 3:00 AM.

- *Telemarketing*—Ads are forever in the trades seeking actors to do sales work. You could be selling long-distance phone service, theatre subscriptions, cable television packages, or spatulas. These jobs offer very flexible schedules and short shifts, late shifts, early shifts, you name it, which means little interference with auditions. It's also a great place to study people and develop characters. The pay is decent, and they usually add a commission. The downside is that you're that annoying person calling people.

T

Television Auditions

Television employment is the bread-and-butter work for most actors in Hollywood. Look at a working actor's resume and you'll see a *TV Guide* of credits. Film and commercial work comes, too, but television is the big employer for the average actor. As such, casting directors for network, syndicated, pay channel, and cable shows are very popular people with performers.

Auditioning for television is usually a two part process—prereads and producer callbacks. Television casting can be brutally fast. A Breakdown can come out for a costar role on a sitcom that is going to be cast by the next day. Thus, there's little time to work extensively on character definition. Actors who are quick on their feet and able to digest new material quickly survive well in television auditions. To be a working actor, you'll learn to do that as well.

I remember one call I got for a sitcom pilot where they phoned me on a Sunday night and said the call was for 9:15 the next morning, and there were no sides available. I arrived to find eight or nine actors who looked just like me waiting at the studio gate for admittance. We were all ushered in, given some hastily prepared sides, and the auditions were over half an hour later. The role was shooting that afternoon, so the need for the rush was pretty obvious.

Most television auditions are not so frenzied, however. Casting directors leave enough time for the actor to get ahold of audition material and work on the part before reading for the role. Twenty-four to forty-eight hours is the most common time frame. This will even afford you ample opportunity to meet with an acting coach to work on the material or at least rehearse at home. Once you've studied the material, somewhat memorized the lines, and figured out the framework, you'll then head to the office to audition.

When you arrive to a television call, you are usually joined by other actors reading for parts as well. The waiting room can be a crowded place on a busy casting day. Each office has its own way of doing this. Some will schedule all the actors reading for the role of "Burt" to come in one after another. Others will stagger each role so that you might not be there when other "Burts" are waiting but will see other actors sign in to read for the parts of "Steve," "Debbie," and "Hank." This can be dictated by the caster's preference or by time constraints.

You may be reading with the casting director or an assistant; more often than not, it will *not* be on-camera, unlike for commercials and sometimes for feature films. In the rare instances that they do tape a television audition, the video cassette will be shot and rushed over to producers and an actor will be booked soon thereafter. More common though is a casual audition, or as casual as an audition can be. Given the enormous pressure casting directors are under to deliver new guest casts week in and week out they do manage to make the auditions pleasant.

How an actor gets to and through the television casting process is explained by casting director Brian Myers. Explains Myers,

> I put out a Breakdown and go through the piles of pictures, and there's always a lot. I'll pull the ones that look appropriate, if I don't know the actors, and set up times for them to come in. If it's somebody I haven't met before I try to talk to them a little bit before we read. For two reasons; I want to learn a little bit more about them and I also want to make them feel comfortable. I don't want them to think this is a pressure situation. You can put too much pressure on yourself. So, we read the scene and if I think they don't have the right take on it I'll give them some notes and we'll try it again. Or if they're great the next step would be to take them over to see the producers. It's sort of the same situation there, but there are more people in the room, and we probably wouldn't chat. I try to discourage chatting because it can work against you. Then the actor does the scene and that's it. Usually, for the callback, I'll bring in six to eight people per role and on occasion if the producers can't make up their mind or they want to see something different we'll have another callback. Then I'll call and negotiate the deal and get them to the set.

Prereads—A preread is the first audition for a television project. It could be a confusing term to a new actor because it implies it's something you are going to do before an actual audition, when in fact it is the audition. It allows the casting director to see a larger number of actors and determine who they want to bring back for the second audition or callback. It's also an excellent way for the caster to meet new talent and see what they can bring to a role. The casting director may also have more time at this juncture to work with you a bit in getting you toward a better or more appropriate performance. There's no time for that later.

Casting director Lisa Miller Katz explains,

> If I have time to do a day of prereads I always do them. I love to do them. If time doesn't permit me to do it then I'm more likely to just

bring in the folks that I really know and trust whose work I'm very familiar with. I'll preread maybe sixty people and show the producers six to eight actors. If it's an actor I know well I'm usually not going to ask for a preread, but if the role is a total one eighty from what I'm used to seeing them do I will ask them to do it. Some actors like that.

In a few casting offices, especially when roles are not dialogue heavy, a preread might not be with the main casting director, but with an associate there. This doesn't change anything about what you do. The associate is the casting director for all intents and purposes. They may be reading with you again if you land a callback, at which time the main caster will almost always be in attendance.

Some experienced actors take offense with prereads, especially if they've previously read or been hired by the casting director in the recent past. Adds Miller Katz, "There are some actors, who if you ask them to preread the agent calls and says, 'Absolutely not, bring her to the producers, you know what she can do.' So every case is individual."

A surviving actor would be well served to put his ego aside and look at the rich possibilities of a preread. Although a casting director will often bring a proven entity directly to the producer, thereby hurdling the preread phase, it could in some cases be a disadvantage. Although undoubtedly pleasing to the actor's self-esteem, he will find himself at the callback with other performers who have preread and who might be more in tune with the part.

At a preread, which in most cases shouldn't be a very hectic affair, the actor often has much more time to work with the casting director on the part. It is not uncommon for there to be two or three go-rounds at the material, if the casting director likes what you are doing. She may give you adjustments as she directs you and will sometimes tell you what the producers are looking for. Without that preread, you might be the only actor of the five called back who doesn't realize the character is supposed to be confused rather than defensive. This one piece of information might be the difference between getting the part and going home to a quiet pager.

So why would you, an actor who wants to survive, at any stage of your career, get upset when you are asked to preread for a casting director who already knows you can act? Let your ego go and know that you are being given two opportunities—to learn something you might not know and to audition in a relative safety zone.

You'll likely encounter three scenarios on prereads. There are some casting directors who preread everyone, whether the actor has worked for them several times before or not at all. Then there are those who'll only preread newer actors or actors they haven't seen in awhile. The third scenario I've encountered is the casting director who is bringing in an actor for a kind of role they haven't seen them do before—perhaps an ingénue reading for a nemesis role or a blue-collar guy for a refined lawyer. It's always nice when this happens.

Each audition has a life of its own, and a lot of it is dictated by the person reading opposite you. Some casting directors are really strong actors in their own right (in fact, many were actors), and will give you a lot with which to work. Others simply read the copy and don't act at all. Expect both in your career, and because you are quick you'll be able to adapt to each situation as it occurs. Some will interact with you completely, and others will barely look up as they read from their own script. Usually, it's something in-between. Whatever the case may be on any given day, give your best read, hit the lines, and maybe you'll be called back to do it for the producers.

Producer Callbacks—Producer callbacks, or simply callbacks, are just another way of saying that this is your second-round television show audition, and they are an eye-opener for actors accustomed to other acting media. Where else are you going to walk into a room that is literally filled with two to twenty people who will all have an opinion (after you've left, thankfully) on whether you should be cast.

By the way, they're referred to as producer calls for two reasons. The producers, who are usually the creators and writers, are going to be there. The director may not. The directors, if they're not working on other episodes, may not even be hired yet. As such, the producers usually make the casting decisions. If a director is in attendance, the casting director will sometimes say something like, "This is our director," when they introduce you to the room. Don't count on it happening too often; otherwise, they'd be referring to these things as producer-director callbacks.

So how do you survive producer calls? First, you should congratulate yourself for having made it this far in the process. The casting director has called you back, after an obviously solid preread, to meet the people who write, produce, and possibly direct the show on which you are hoping to appear. That's a great thing—well done. You nailed it, but the job isn't yours, yet. Now when they call your name, the real work begins.

Depending on the casting director and producer's preference, there will be anywhere from a few actors to maybe a dozen brought in at callback for each role. Rest assured, it won't be as many as auditioned at the preread. It's usually a reasonable number. You'll be ushered into the casting room, which is almost always a different location than where you had your first audition, to read for the creative team. They are almost always supportive and a great audience, even after they've sat through an abundance of actors doing the same material.

You'll see a lot of unfamiliar faces at the same moment. Don't try to meet everyone individually. A general "hello" to the room will suffice; don't rush over to them to shake hands—it takes too much time. Read the room. Although the casting rule of thumb is to come in and get right to the material, if someone there engages you in conversation or jumps up to shake your hand then go with it. But remember to follow their lead.

Most of the time you'll walk into the room, the casting director or assistant will announce your name, and you'll discover a slew of smiling faces. There's usually an obvious place to stand; if not, just pick one, a fair distance from the audience, as you prepare to do your reading with either the assistant or the CD. It's almost always the same person you read with at the preread.

You'll get into your audition, and you'll probably want to do it just like you did the first time. The casting director's endorsement by bringing you back has told you this. Doing it the same is easier said than done. It's always going to be somewhat new. Your intention may be to do it the same, but your whole delivery might change if you start off on a different beat than you did before. Go with it. It's better to create fresh than try to fight your way back and find an old performance. Even if you are doing it somewhat differently, you can still find enough of the right beats throughout to keep it in the same range as what got you the callback.

If you get off on a bad foot, stop yourself and ask graciously if you can start again. They will always say "yes." However, this only applies to the first four or five lines. Once you're further into it, push on even if you get off base. Don't worry about missing a line or not hitting it as well as you did in the preread. If you're the right type, if they like you, and if you get most of it in the ballpark, you have a shot. Even better is you'll repeat the magic you brought to the first read and maybe even step it up a notch, and then it's up to them to make their decision.

Most of the time, after you read, you'll get more smiling and the casting director or one of the producers will say "thank you." That's your cue to leave. Say "thank you" and don't feel the need to kiss up to everyone. They've seen it all before, and they don't like it. Leave the way you came in and get home so you can start sending out more pictures.

On occasion, they won't excuse you so fast. Now you'll definitely find out who is the head honcho. He will ask you to do it again, but they'll give you a little adjustment. This is good news. It means you are a real contender for the part. But you'd better make the adjustment, because if you repeat the read you just gave, they may think you weren't paying attention or can't take direction. You don't usually get a chance to do it again in television (it's much more common in film auditions) because of the pace and because callbacks are scheduled so that all actors are there at once. They must keep these sessions moving.

Test Deals

Test deals are the contracts you sign before you get to the final rung of auditioning for a series regular role. That's right, *before*. No pressure there, huh?

Test deals send shivers down the spine. They're great because they mean you are oh-so-close to landing a regular role on a new, or sometimes, existing television series. You are literally at the last step before getting what could turn out to be the dream job.

But here's the rub. It's not intimidating enough that you are going to strut your stuff in front of the network suits—the president, vice president's studio executives, and all manner of creative forces behind those big-budget television hits. Prior to walking into the room, before you read one word for the people who will collectively voice their opinion on your talent, your likeability, and maybe your hair color, you will be asked to sign a big-time contract.

That's the way it works when you are trying to land a starring role in television. It starts out with the preread, then on to the producers, who may want you to audition several times before they schedule the test sessions in front of the brass—first at the studio level and then at the network. They negotiate the terms of your contract upfront, just in case you book the part. When actors audition for guest work on shows, their contracts are done after the booking. But for the performers at this level, the producers want all the Is dotted, Ts crossed, and appropriate numbers filled in. Do you tempt fate and even read the thing? Well, you have to, but then you'd better get it out of your system so you can go in and read without that baggage on your back. Test deals are done beforehand to ensure the producers that an actor won't try to get more money than is in the budget once everyone is in agreement that this is *the* actor for the part.

Caster Lisa Miller Katz goes more in-depth on the subject:

> When we are going to test an actor, I'll call the agent and tell them that business affairs from the studio will be calling to make a test option deal, and that will determine your salary and what the raises will be every year and what the billing will be. All of the specifics are negotiated. Then I'm assigned a time when I'm testing all the actors reading for the role of "Joe," so I bring in maybe six people to the studio casting people and executives and they pick their favorites. The best of the bunch go onto the network people, the President, V.P.'s, etc. and re-audition again. You're talking about fifteen to twenty people in the room when you read. There's a lot of different opinions and it can be very intimidating.

Breathe deep, count your lucky stars, and remember that most actors never get the chance to do a test deal. You are doing very well.

Theatre in Los Angeles

Los Angeles is truly becoming a city in which actors can find serious theatre opportunity, but I'd be remiss if I didn't tell it like it really is. Even though there is certainly a significant theatre scene—numberswise one of the largest in the world—and one that is vociferously defended by its creators, the stage still takes a big back seat to the sound stage.

In this continually evolving stage scene, theatre is now starting to be regarded for theatre's sake and, in the last few years, there has been an emergence of some world-class ensemble companies that you might think fell through the earth in Greenwich Village and emerged somewhere near downtown LA.

Rob Kendt, the Editor in Chief/Associate Publisher of *Backstage West* has about as much knowledge as anyone in Los Angeles on the local and, for that matter, national, theatre scene. His trade paper covers the scene extensively, and Kendt has been known to make an appearance as an actor and/or musician in productions. His comments accurately reflect the way the scene is currently looking.

Kendt explains,

> Theatre isn't an industry in Los Angeles, it's more of a community of artists, working mostly in non-paying or low-paying venues just to keep acting and doing their art (and, in part, for the purpose of showing their work to film and TV industry folks). That said, there has been significant growth in prestige, quality, and reputation of the LA theatre scene, and the audience has grown accordingly—which means also that there has been an encouraging increase in the number of local Equity contracts, as well as local auditions for big national stage productions. Bottom line, LA is a place actors come to pursue film and TV careers, not theatre careers—but it's become a place where actors increasingly find they don't have to give up doing meaty, creatively satisfying stage work while they're busy playing the Hollywood lottery and waiting for the phone to ring.

The biggest theatre *employer*, although that's stretching the term, for actors here is the AEA ninety-nine-seat plan, which allows Equity members and nonunion actors to work for just a few dollars per performance in certain theatres with ninety-nine or less seating capacity.

Fueling the growth of the local scene are the larger resident companies such as A Noise Within, East West Players, and the Will Geer Theatricum Botanicum and premiere ninety-nine-seat companies such as the Odyssey Theatre Ensemble, Matrix Theatre Company, Deaf West Theatre, and Actor's Gang. There are also numerous quality membership companies, comedy/improv troupes, excellent mid-size theatres such as the Mark Taper Forum, Geffen Playhouse, and El Portal Theatre, and a few Broadway style houses such as the Ahmanson and the Pantages, which offer major League of Resident Theatre (LORT) contracts.

Los Angeles theatre has struggled somewhat because of the film and television business, but not solely for that reason. The city's size has also hurt it, but even that's changing. Too often, it's been hard to draw consistent audiences to anything other than the biggest shows. Many people aren't willing to drive five miles, let alone twenty, to see a production. But more recently there seems to be something in the air.

Due primarily to those resident and independent companies that put on consistently stellar work, Angelenos are increasingly making the trek to the theatre more often and supporting live theatre that *doesn't* have a singing lion with ticket purchases or subscription commitments. Revitalized areas such as the North Hollywood Arts District are theatre intensive and easily accessible, which also encourages more patronage. Various factors are conspiring to make this a theatre town. Now, if they can just get those ninety-nine-seat contracts for actors up a few notches, things will really start to soar.

With all this theatre going on, would you come here today *solely* to make a living as a stage actor? That's a tough call, due to the financial aspects, but you can certainly find solid opportunities to do quality theatre, not just the industry showcase version so well-known to Los Angeles. This has been the biggest change in the last ten years, and now LA can legitimately claim itself a real theatre town. Between nationally recognized companies, revitalized theatre districts, a growing number of festivals, and the national touring shows, which hold local auditions here a few times per year, Los Angeles performers can indeed see themselves beyond just the lens of a camera.

Tracking

What is tracking? It's the way you stay on top of people who have hired, auditioned, directed, aided, or in any way helped you to further your career. Tracking is staying in touch, following up, and keeping the lines of communication open—all rolled into one.

Tracking starts by keeping a log of all auditions, appointments, meetings, mailings, and connections you've made. I'm not suggesting you need to keep a physical record of every encounter you have in your daily career, although some actors do just that. But I will suggest you take notes of the better experiences and build on them from those tracking records. Believe me, you'll need them.

It goes beyond mere marketing and focuses on building on genuine industry contacts who already know you. It's one thing to do a

mass mailing, and you'll certainly have some of those during your career, but it's another thing to stay in touch with someone with whom
you've actually established some kind of a professional relationship.
Let's say you read for a casting director but didn't get that particular
role, yet she mentioned that she'd like to see you in something on
stage. You'd better take that note down, add it to your tracking log, and
take her up on it later. What sounds like a better approach to you—"Hi,
I'm appearing in . . . " or "Hi, you mentioned you'd like to see me in a
stage production. I'll be appearing next week . . . "? Keep track of the
moments that have substance. After an audition, if a casting director
says, "I'll be seeing you," it's not the same as "I'd like to have you in
to read again sometime." Try to be objective and track the things that
have the highest potential for payoff.

Although tracking can be tedious and unglamorous, the results can
pay off in dividends. By tracking, you are keeping your mind active
and focused on your career. Maybe it's not playing a role, but you are
being proactive, laying the groundwork to get you on that next set. It
can actually be kind of fun if you don't fight it too much. Anything that
takes your mind off your silent pager is a good thing.

There is another more defined level of tracking; keeping in contact
with those people with whom you've genuinely established a *working*
relationship. You'd also better have a list of your bookings. Nothing
would be worse than forgetting that a casting director was nice enough
to book you three years earlier. If you hit it off with a director on set,
you'd be foolish to waste that opportunity for future contact. When a
producer takes you aside and says he likes your work and wants to have
you back again for another episode, you should then track his progress
through the trades.

Hollywood is a publicity town and it's not hard to follow others'
careers. Read the trades, pay attention to the film and television listings, and keep an eye on the Web for new productions. You'll start to
see the names of the people with whom you've already established relationships or worked for. This is your database. When that person is
casting, hiring, or directing a project and you're right for it, follow up at
the opportune time. What sounds better here, "I'd welcome the opportunity to read for your film . . . " or "It was a pleasure working with you
two years ago. I've heard about your new project and feel I'd be perfect
for the role of . . . ". You see the difference? It's just smart connecting,
but many actors don't take the time to do it.

Let me give you an example of superb tracking. A friend of mine
played a wonderful role in a blockbuster film in the early 1990s. He
heard about the project early on, did some research, and probably knew
about the same time as the regional casting director that they were going
to be using local hires for some of the roles. A few months later he had

a part and found himself working with one of the top directors in the business.

After the first film wrapped, the actor made it a point to keep track of the director, the producer, and their projects. A few times a year, he sent them postcards announcing things he'd booked or was appearing in. Nothing inappropriately aggressive—just enough to keep him on their radar for the future. Eventually, he heard about another project the director was doing and wrote to him, via the production company, and soon enough the director hired him for another nice role. The producer from the first film later gave his name to another producer who hired him for yet a third project.

That's a big-time tracking success story. Would the actor have gotten a part in that second film if he'd just let the ball drop, not kept up on that particular director, or not known that he was returning to that area to shoot another film? Would the impression he'd made four years earlier been strong enough for the helmer to remember him without the benefit of getting those postcards three or four times per year? Would the producer recommendation have happened by osmosis? I doubt it. There are a lot of good actors available. That actor took the guess work out of the equation. If he didn't get any more work from them, it wouldn't have been for lack of trying.

Tracking might not lead directly to repeated acting jobs or even a job, but it will make you a much better informed actor. Here's another variety of nonbooking tracking that any auditioning actor can use. You've auditioned for a show and the casting director gives you a note, perhaps telling you that the pacing needs to be faster. When you go home, you put that information in your tracking notes, because chances are if the caster wanted you to pick up the pace on that audition he'll probably want the same the next time he reads you for that same show. If you have any doubts, maybe they're erased when you read an interview with the casting director in *Backstage West* where he states that the producer of the show he's casting likes actors who are adept at rapid-fire dialogue. That's the same note twice, and you'll certainly remember it the next time out because you kept a record.

You don't have to track. You can just wait it out, do an occasional general mailing, and see where the chips fall, but will you be doing the most you can for your acting career?

Traffic

LA's traffic is legendary. It's massive, intimidating, and relentless, and it's also been blown somewhat out of proportion. The fact is, if you've come from almost any major metropolitan area, you are already familiar with sitting in traffic jams, overheating engines, and being a few minutes late for work. Just multiply it a few times and you'll understand the LA wheel deal.

Everybody drives in LA, and very few car pool. The inevitable result are a lot of vehicles squeezing onto freeways that were designed when there were half as many cars and many fewer actors. And no one drives more than an actor. You'll spend a good part of your life in LA zipping between Hollywood and the Valley and back again to the Westside and east to downtown. You will learn to navigate like a New York cabbie.

Speaking of New York hacks; let me tell you about an actor I know who used to drive a cab in Manhattan. He moved to LA a few years before me, and when I arrived gave me a few excellent tips about surviving the driving scene. He took me around and actually showed me this on the streets. I'll share these survival tips with you.

Number one, he said, was to stay off anything that looks like a ramp to a freeway from 3:00 PM to around 7:00 PM. The freeways are no actor's land during those hours and must be avoided, especially if you are heading to an audition. You will be late.

Now, in the eight years I've lived here, I've learned something. Traffic has gotten that much worse. I've discussed this matter in-depth with friends and we're all pretty much in agreement that freeways should be avoided anytime you can avoid them. At 11:00 PM, you're pretty safe, but if you can find a surface road that'll almost always be your saving grace. There are times during business hours when the freeways are wide open, but it's rare. Or it might appear to be wide open until you head over the hill and suddenly you're facing a thousand red taillights and your audition is in five minutes. Be careful about that, and stick to the surface streets when you can.

There are a ton of alternate routes to just about everywhere. Actors learn these routes out of sheer survival, which leads me to that second piece of wisdom my cabbie pal shared. LA drivers are notoriously loyal to their favorite routes. Let's say someone has a survival job in Santa Monica and lives in midcity, which is several miles away. This driver may prefer to take his cross route trip via Olympic Boulevard. He'll do that day in and day out. Sounds okay; it's direct. But what do you do when things are tied up? Most drivers in most cities would find another street. For some reason, the actor told me, in many cases they just don't do that here. But as a smarty, you will.

To prove his point, he took me around town on surface streets and we came upon two very busy and slow-moving traffic situations. We sat in these jams for ten minutes or so to prove the point, and then he said, "Now let me show you something." He made a quick right, went over one block, and made a left onto the next major street. Voila, no traffic! We rode merrily and traffic free for twenty minutes before crossing back over to the original street. Miles away and it was still blocked. Commuters were locked into their favorite street. Don't do it. Producers are waiting on you, and gas costs too much.

Turning Down Work

Most of the time turning down work isn't an option when you are an average actor. Most of us don't have studios sending us scripts with back-end participation deals locked in; nor do we have drivers picking us up for our 5:00 AM calls. When a job is offered, even one that's a pretty lousy role, you usually take it.

Some roles make you a better actor, some pay the bills, and some just get you working again, which makes you all the much more prepared for that better role that you hope is right around the corner. Short of porn, if you're a surviving actor, you take the job that's offered.

But every so often you have to stop and take a real close look at something that doesn't feel right. There could be a lot of reasons for this—you don't like the content of the material, the pay rate isn't anywhere near your quote rate, or it's a location shoot in Guam and you don't fly. Maybe they want you to do a stunt. If that's the case, you do what's right for you. You don't live and die by one job, and don't let anyone tell you that you do.

Maybe you'll say "no" to one because something just goes against your own personal belief system. I used to smoke. As a matter of fact, when I take my trip or two to Vegas each year, I still have been known to bum one from someone at the Blackjack table. I should know better. My mother died of breast cancer.

About a year after she passed away, I was called in for a commercial audition for a German tobacco company. They were doing a spoof of American stereotypes—the macho cowboy, the gung-ho military guy (my part), and several other stereotypical roles. While waiting for my time to read, I finally started to think about what this was really about. It was about smoking. Did I really want to promote smoking to teenagers, even if they were in Dusseldorf instead of Detroit? My wonderful mom had suffered greatly. But wait, what a hypocrite I was being. It was okay for me to have the occasional cigarette but draw a line in the sand and not do a commercial for a company whose product I occasionally used? I was bothered by the whole thing, but I wasn't bothered enough to walk away from the call.

I did the audition and then signed out. I went home and got a call from my agent sometime later. They wanted to put me on avail. That's a nice Hollywood way of saying, we like you and may want to book you so don't leave town on these dates or we'll never hire you again. It does not mean they have hired you.

So I was momentarily happy and then the whole thought process started up anew. This time ethics won out over the need for cash. After a few hours, I called my agent to tell her that I wasn't available for those dates. I didn't even get into the real reason until a later conversation when I told her I never wanted to be submitted for a tobacco project again. After I made the decision, I never looked back and now it's so clear to me that I could never do that kind of ad. I'm glad I live in America where it's not the most difficult decision, as tobacco ads are nonexistent on television. It would be really tough if I had something against cereal.

There's a more common method of turning down work that has nothing to do with role content but role size. Many actors have decided that they aren't playing costars when they have been getting hired as guest stars. In the credit-building and quote-establishing world of film and television, it's not always just about the work. As such, people are sometimes forced to decide on the job based on what it might do to them perceptionwise in the industry. A costarring role, which might be a few lines to pages of dialogue, is a wonderful gig for most actors, but once you've gotten to the next rung on the ladder it might not be an offer you want. Each actor and their talent representatives have to decide the game plan and when they are willing to deviate from it.

Casting director Lisa Miller Katz notes,

> For every actor who says to me I don't want to do costarring roles, I can tell you of twenty others who are in danger of losing their insurance. If you don't want to do it, there are plenty of people who need it more. An actor has to decide at a certain point what price he's willing to pay to not get a job. And this happens to casting directors as well.

Typecasting

If you are going to be an actor in Hollywood, you'd better get used to the fact that you will often be typecast. Typecasting gets a bad rap, but the fact of the real acting business is that it's not such a bad thing. It means you are getting hired. If getting an acting job and a paycheck is the price for being typecast, well, they can type away as far as this actor is concerned. Although no one loves the idea of it, many of the busiest actors are typed. If you get typed enough, hired enough, and achieve some leverage in the business, you can eventually move beyond it.

Agent Patty Grana-Miller explains,

> It is what it is. When a project, whether it be a commercial, motion picture or TV show is being cast they have determined what they want for each role based on a lot of factors, and that usually can't be

changed. We try to push the envelope whenever we can—sometimes it works and sometimes it doesn't.

You can stop getting yourself typecast by changing your type. Grow a beard, lose fifty pounds, start pumping iron, have a facelift—there are a million ways to change your type, but you know what happens then? You just become another type and get typecast as that. You've only traded in one type for another. Film and television are often about appearance, so typecasting is an inevitable reality.

No actor wants to go through years of playing only one type of role, but that's exactly how many performers established themselves before becoming bigger players, and then breaking out of their type because of their stature. That's the leverage. As any shrewd performer will attest, there are a wide range of roles within each type and you always try to make the role go beyond the written type. Casting is a fast and first-impression business. There isn't a lot of time to intellectualize why an actor who is physically against type should be brought before a producer. It happens, but it's the exception. They want that first image to convey a feeling. That guy is a thug, this one's the hero, and she's the femme fatale.

If you are absolutely appalled by typecasting, then you should avoid Hollywood. In fact, you should avoid the film industry altogether because it isn't going to change. Let them type you. Make your resume and reel grow, work your way up the established ranks, then you might be able to overcome it. Then again, you may not and still have a fantastic career. I can think of five well-known actors who are B-level players who have been playing type for decades. That's five amazing careers by five survivors. You should be so lucky as to be typed because it sure beats being an out-of-work actor.

U

Unemployment

Unemployment is all too often the real full-time occupation of the surviving actor. Working is the part-time part. Unfortunately, you aren't compensated for that part of your career. You'll need to find some way to supplement your annual income during those down times.

The federal government comes to the rescue! Unemployment works a little differently for professional actors than it does for most other occupational workers, in that it is common to see actors go on and off unemployment insurance several times per year. Assuming you've earned at least $1300 in a three-month period here in California, even from a single day of work on a show, you will usually be able to avail yourself of benefits for a minimum of six months. Hopefully, you've worked more than that or your payment will probably be very low.

The Employment Development Department bases your benefits on a three-month cycle. There are four cycles per year in which you can be eligible, and they'll determine your payment based on your highest earnings quarter. So if you've worked one job in one three-month period and made $600 but worked eight jobs in a subsequent three-month period earning $6000, they'll base your weekly amount on the higher quarter. This is especially attractive to actors who find themselves earning in wild swings throughout the years.

If you haven't been here long enough to get benefits, you are eligible to receive benefits from your former state and then transition into the California plan once you have earned money here. So let's say you came here from New York City where you worked extensively last year. If you haven't done any acting work in LA, you'd apply through the New York office. It's all done federally so the different offices will coordinate fairly well. You claim through New York and collect until those benefits run out. In the meantime, you get as much work as you can in LA and then you'll reapply for benefits in California at a later date.

Now here's where it gets a bit trickier. Actors go on and off unemployment all the time. Here's how it works in a nutshell. Let's say you're collecting $200 per week in unemployment and you've landed an acting gig on a television show. The job pays you $700 for the day.

On your unemployment form, you'll mark down the date that you were employed, who the employer of record was (employer of record because payroll firms that work for the producers are usually identified as the employer), and the amount they paid you. You'll also note on the form that your employment was completed because you were hired and have already finished your duties for that project.

When your next biweekly check arrives (each unemployment check is for two pay weeks), you will not get benefits for one of the two weeks because you worked. However, you don't *lose* that week's benefit, it is just pushed back a week so that you can claim it on your next form. In other words, you aren't penalized for having gotten a job. When you originally applied for benefits, they would have told you your total benefit amount and you'll get that amount in full. It might be paid out in six months (if you don't land any work during that time), or it might take you a full year to exhaust your benefits, assuming you've landed several days of work during that six-month period). I guess this nutshell is pretty big, because there's more. Let's now assume you didn't actually work but still received a residual check in the mail for an old acting job. You still mark that down as money earned. Depending on the amount of the residual, you will either get no employment benefit for that week or a partial benefit. This is exhausting, but we're almost done.

If you're a working actor, you'll be able to open up a whole new claim again once your next filing period arrives, which will be exactly one year after the first one started. Now, when you do hit the acting level where you get a full-time job, perhaps a series regular or an extended film or theatre commitment, you will be glad to mark off on your last claim form that you no longer need the benefits because you are employed for the foreseeable future. That will be a very good day.

Unions

To survive in Hollywood, you're eventually going to need to be in at least two unions—SAG and AFTRA. These two organizations collectively represent the acting talent for virtually all major programs on television, in film, and on the radio. If you emptied the airwaves of all the union talent on any given night, viewers at home would be watching shows with wonderful sets but devoid of humans. The unions are where you, the actor, must be one day if you plan on surviving as a professional performer.

Here's the rundown on the unions:

- *Screen Actors Guild, 5757 Wilshire Boulevard, Los Angeles, CA 90036-3600, phone: 523-954-1600*—There are about 98,600 SAG members in the United States. According to SAG, approximately 59,000 are here in the Los Angeles region. SAG members are principal on-camera actors, voice-over talent, stunt performers, background artists, and even pilots who fly their planes through shots. SAG has all the films, primetime dramas, and most of the half-an-hour comedies to call their own. Previously, the rule of thumb was that if it is shot on film, it's covered by SAG. If it's shot on tape, it's covered by AFTRA. That's still pretty accurate, although there are some programs done on tape that still fall under SAG's jurisdiction.

SAG does not get work for actors, but instead negotiates contracts, oversees working conditions, processes residual payments, and deals with agencies that represent its members. This last point is in flux. As of mid-2002, the long-term agreement between SAG and the ATA ended, after a hotly contested battle which resulted in SAG's membership voting down a new agreement. By the time you're reading this book, we all hope there is further clarification on these issues. To be safe, call SAG if you have agency questions. As of July 2002, SAG's actors were still working with their formerly franchised ATA agents, since SAG has put a temporary suspension on Rule 16—which requires actors to be represented only by a franchised agent.

SAG is not an open union, so you must meet certain requirements to join. Once you are a member, you can no longer do nonunion work, but you are now a part of the world's most powerful performing arts organization.

- *AFTRA, 5757 Wilshire Boulevard, Suite 900, Los Angeles, CA 90036, phone: 323-634-8100*—This union covers daytime soap operas, live and taped variety programs such as *"The Tonight Show,"* radio shows and spots, newscasts, and some taped sitcoms. AFTRA has 90,000 members nationally and about 30,000 around LA. AFTRA takes a bit of a back seat in this SAG-dominated village, but it is a remarkably well-run union and works extremely well with SAG, even though the long talked-about merger between the two performers' organizations was royally kyboshed a few years back. Nevertheless, they remain *good friends* and share the same business address, although on different floors. AFTRA is an open union, which means anyone with the initiation fee who wants to call themself an AFTRA member may do so after first visiting the office and turning over a check. AFTRA does the same things for its members that SAG does for theirs. Many members, in fact, are in both of these unions.

Both SAG and AFTRA have excellent health plans, decent pension plans, a shared credit union, casting information hotlines, newsletters, occasional agent/casting director showcases, and other programs for their members. What they don't often have is enough work.

Even though joining the unions is a necessity for most long-term actors, doing so is no guarantee of success or even employment. Statistics don't lie. According to SAG, about seventy percent of their members make less than $9000 a year. Fifteen to twenty percent make somewhere between $9000 and $50,000 annually. Given the ups and down of being an actor, you might make $9000 one year, $20,000 the next, and $5000 the following year. Try to do family budget with that kind of salary swing. Eight to ten percent earn over $50,000, and only two percent make more than $250,000. These numbers come directly from SAG in March 2002, and vary slightly from those reported elsewhere, but they are clear in showing that very few working actors are living on easy street and most are making well below a liveable wage.

- *Actors' Equity Association, 5757 Wilshire Boulevard, Los Angeles, CA 90036, phone: 323-634-1750*—There is another major union in town and that is AEA. It's a tremendous union of stage performers that you might or might not ever need to join in Los Angeles. The reason is the lion's share of professional theater falls under the AEA ninety-nine-seat plan, which allows union and nonunion stage actors to work together for a few bucks per performance.

You don't need to be in AEA to do these shows, but if you have higher theatrical aspirations than ninety-nine-seaters alone, an AEA card should be in your plan. Some of the resident theatre companies require it for auditions, but a nonunion actor has a much better chance of being seen after AEA principal auditions than he would in New York.

As the larger theatre scene grows and more substantive contracts are offered, AEA membership will become a more attractive option for actors and stage managers who are also covered under the union's jurisdiction. As this occurs, more people will undoubtedly follow their New York brethren and find their way into the AEA membership rolls of 45,000. In the meantime, a lot of ninety-nine-seat theatre producers are getting top-notch talent for the price of a burger combo at McDonald's.

V

Victim Mentality

No one in that office will hire me.
That casting director doesn't like me.
I've paid my dues, why should I have to read for that part?
I can't get an agent because I'm too old.
SAG actors get all the good jobs.
I don't look like a supermodel, so I don't get auditions.

This is an unfair business sometimes. Accept it and don't make it worse by falling into the role of victim. If you become a professional complainer, it weakens you. Negativity feeds on itself, and before you know it you're spending even more time talking about what's not working for you and how Hollywood is out to get you. Eventually, that's all that remains. For every one of these victim statements, and for all the others that exist, there are several solutions. Survivors find them.

So if there's a casting director who doesn't like you, think about the other three hundred with whom you don't have that problem. If one office won't bring you in, do a mailing to the others who might. If you've paid your dues, pay them again; they don't owe you anything. If an agent thinks you're too old, remember that *twenty* is too old and find another agent.

Attitude is everything in this business. If you feel good, then you will do good. If you walk around like the world is weighing you down, then no one is going to want to work with you. There are actors all over town like this. There are also other actors who haven't worked in months who you'd think just hit the lottery. They have. They just haven't gotten the payoff yet.

Voice-Over Work

Everything you've heard about voice work is true. Employment is hard to get, a relative few dominate in the field, and it's very expensive to try to even join the fold. Between proper training, which you must have before ever venturing into this field, and the cost of making a professional demo produced by an engineer who knows the current marketplace—you are talking about thousands of dollars and many months of education.

The bottom line is that voice work is a full-time commitment on its own. If you're going to pursue it, go for it, but do so with a game plan or you'll be throwing your money away and potentially taking time away from your on-camera acting endeavors. However, and most voice artists will tell you this, if you are committed to the craft, the area is not an impenetrable fortress. You'll just need your best weapons.

Voice-over isn't just about having a great voice. It's about having an extremely versatile voice and being a great actor who can nail the role without the benefit of visual physicality to help to portray the part. It's all done from the throat, and there's no camera to catch your great reaction shots. You have to be able to do audio copy over and over, hit beats, make quick adjustments when the client demands them, and get it in at the exact same time frame repeatedly. The known voice-over actors are a very talented bunch—the ultimate cold readers, as they may read five, ten, or more characters per day while auditioning. Those are numbers an on-camera actor couldn't imagine in his best week or even month.

Bob Bergen has those numbers and more. A prolific voice actor in Los Angeles, he has done hundreds of commercials, cartoons, and films. He's been the voice of Porky, Tweety, and Marvin the Martian in "Space Jam." He also teaches an animation voice-over class in Los Angeles. Let him tell you more about how these voice-overs work:

> The steps for getting into voice-over are, study to the point where you are ready to make a demo, make the demo, get an agent, start auditioning and get work. Is it that easy? Of course not. Most actors want to take one or two classes, make a demo and take their chances. But one bad demo will ruin a whole career. If your demo isn't top notch it'll be very hard to get your next one listened to. You'll need to take all kinds of classes with a variety of teachers. Don't take a voice-over class if you've had no acting training or experience. You will be taking your acting skills and using them for voice-over. So, how do you know when you're ready for a demo? You just know. It's pure confidence that you can give a competitive read to any piece of copy without spending a lot of time to prepare. Getting an agent is the hardest part of the process. There are hundreds of theatrical and on-camera agents in Los Angeles, but there are only twenty voice-over agents! Getting a voice-over agent is harder than getting a voice-over job. The best way is to have someone in the biz refer you, but the good agents listen to every demo submitted. After the first 4–10 seconds an agent knows if you have what it takes or not. And if an agent passes, and you're good, it's usually because they have someone like you already in their stable. Now, let's say that you got that agent. You should be reading at least 1–3 times a week, sometimes more sometimes less, depending

on how busy the business is in your category. If you aren't working, you should still be in class. You don't want your audition to be your workout. I'll end with this; if you are brilliant, you will work.

Brilliant is quite a ways off from beginning, so you'd be wise to put a lot of time into learning just as you have for your on-camera and theatre work before getting into the business side. When you finally do reach that level, you'll find you're auditioning right at your agent's place of business instead of a casting office. Most of the top voice agents have their own mini sound studios or booths in-house for their talent to come in and lay down the audition. When you're newer, you probably won't have that luxury and will read in the casters' offices. Because this is voice-over, you will see your copy for the first time only when you arrive. You may have only a few minutes to look at the copy. These are fast and the coldest of cold reads. One thing is for sure, there won't be a callback. They hire right from the tapes.

W

Waiting Rooms

Audition waiting rooms are where you'll hang out with your fellow actors before you are called in to show your stuff. They can be fairly cool places with a bunch of professional thespians chatting and being generally supportive of one another. But as any actor will tell you, there is another kind of waiting room, too. This environment can offer an atmosphere of nervous energy, intensity, curiosity, and sometimes outright competition. The audition itself doesn't start until the casting director brings you into her office, but you can very well knock yourself out of the block before you get that far if you allow the waiting room to play with your head too much.

Casting director Lisa Miller Katz has seen what actors sometimes must deal with before they go in to read:

> Sometimes the waiting room can be kind of an icky place. I think you have to learn to focus inward and not sit in the room and compare yourself to other people or listen to everything. There can be a lot of head trips. There may be someone who says something and they could make you feel insecure or bad.

Actress Rosa Fernandez has experienced that uneasy feeling first-hand while waiting to be called in and has figured out a solution that works for her:

> That's one of the things that drives me batty. People start chatting up a storm about anything and everything and sometimes it's not necessarily stuff that you need to hear before you go into an audition. Another thing is when you walk in the waiting room everybody checks you out, everybody checks everybody out. So what I try to do is find a spot kind of away from the brouhaha by myself and try to stay focused until I'm called in.

I've used that method myself. If the pressure gets too much at one of those producer callbacks, you can usually step outside to get a breath of fresh air. Just make sure you check how far down the list your name is so you're actually there to audition when they call your name.

If you find yourself in a positive room with good people, you'll appreciate it and maybe join in the banter. Do whatever works for you, but be cautious about draining too much of your energy before you go into that room to read.

Watching the Show

It amazes me that some actors actually brag that they don't watch television. C'mon! This is your industry and you'd better watch something or you might end up never getting invited to a set to work. I'm not speaking to that thespian debate about *real* actors working in theatre. That's nonsense—a good actor is a good actor, whatever the medium. A smart actor in Hollywood watches where he works. It's called research.

I'm not suggesting that simply watching television is the key to your survival, but it's a big piece of the puzzle and a great gift dropped right in your lap if you know what and when to watch. By viewing programs for which you have a shot at eventually auditioning, you get a sense of what they look for in their guest casts. You pick up on the pacing and style of the show, the manner in which the cast plays their parts, and the overall feel of the operation.

I quickly learned to pay attention to certain shows just as soon as I fouled up early in my first year here. I had an audition for one of those sci-fi shows where the guest and costar aliens all sound vaguely like they are playing Shakespeare. I would have known that if I watched it once. Physically, I was perfect for the part. I'm tall and had a shaved head, and they wanted a menacing type. I could do the menacing thing. I didn't need to watch the show to play mean. So I went in and gave a good reading, or so I thought. What I did wrong was to read the part like some tough guy from Jersey. My approach would have been right on for a cop show but not for one that takes place in another galaxy where everyone has seen Hamlet at least twice. If I'd done my proper research, I would have employed a nice Mid-Atlantic dialect with a dash of a more theatrical delivery. It might have led to a callback. By watching one or two episodes of the show, which I did *afterward,* I could have easily seen the similarity in delivery by the guest cast. I learned from that early error and now pay attention to shows I might be seen for. Surviving actors in LA usually adopt that routine.

Focus a couple of hours per week on shows that traditionally hire actors of your type and age. This strategy of being a career viewer, not just a casual television watcher, has thankfully paid off throughout the years. Case in point: A one-hour drama that I read for that takes place in a certain gritty East Coast city. I watched a couple of episodes and without taxing my brain saw two things. The costars were fairly intense and many were using dialects. At the audition, I used the appropriate regional accent and also punched up the character's intensity a bit more than it read on the page.

Got the job. Did it have anything to do with the passable accent and intensity? I'll never know, but the possibility seemed likelier if I approached it that way. When you feel likelier to succeed, great things can sometimes happen. Even getting one job because you did your homework by watching the show is reason enough to do it. There's no panacea. You could do your due diligence for ten programs and ten auditions, and never even get past the preread. But you might get the eleventh one. The actor who doesn't turn on the set is at a decided disadvantage.

Working Out

True, your body might survive longer if you work out, but that doesn't necessarily mean it'll make you a better actor. Then again, most of the better performances I've seen have been from living actors. You won't be the first actor who moves to Los Angeles who decides to reshape his body, drop a bunch of weight, or suddenly decide, 'Hey, how have I managed to live for thirty years without ever running a marathon?'

Maybe it's the weather, or perhaps it's just because everyone looks so damn good out here, but it's almost inevitable that you will spend some time enhancing your physical self, and that's a good thing for you personally and for your career.

The problem can come in if you start focusing on one over the other. You came here to act—not to compete in the Mr. Manhattan Beach Bikini contest. If you're not focused on your acting first, then it could be easy to get distracted by the ever-present body-enhancing atmosphere of living in Southern California.

Stay in shape, but don't forget your purpose for being here. There are actors in Los Angeles who spend five days a week at the gym toning their abs and building up their guns, yet they couldn't find an acting class if they tripped over one. Some actors have memberships to tanning salons, yoga centers, and pay weekly visits to the chiropractor, but haven't done even a day's extra work or sought out a new photo since the 1980s.

Keep your eye on the ball. Take that acting class and also keep yourself healthy. You'll be a lot happier, not to mention a much better actor, in the long run.

X,Y,&Z

X-Rated

Don't do pornography if you have serious aspirations as an actor. This is in no way a judgment of people who are porn performers. Nevertheless, for someone who plans on being in more traditional Hollywood fare (i.e., the kind where you're not having real sex on-camera), you'd be taking an incredibly short-sighted career view if you think you can do a smoker or two and not have anyone notice.

Southern California is the mecca to not only the television and film industry, but also a hot-bed (literally) of adult entertainment, especially in the San Fernando Valley. There are even talent agencies for porn performers. There are also a lot of attractive young girls and guys who really want to be on-camera, but there's only so much work available. Some end up trying this other kind of entertainment.

There have been one or two cases where people have made somewhat of a cross-over, but it is more likely that a porn career is followed by more porn, not guest star appearances on network television or for roles in legitimate films. Think about where you want to be in ten years.

You, the Boss of You

So I've served up a bunch of advice in this book. That's also what I do in "Tombudsman," and being a Libra apparently has something astrologically to do with that. On occasion, I even listen to my own advice, and sometimes I don't. I do something at an audition or while working or marketing that I haven't done before. I free form, take a chance, go against the grain, live on the edge, or the semi-edge. Sometimes it works and sometimes I go home with my tail between my legs.

Here's why. I'm my own boss. And so are you, my fellow actor. You're the boss of you. You report to you. You give you your assignments and you watch over your performance. Ultimately, you are the CEO (Chief Everything Officer) of your career.

What that means is that, although there is certainly advice to be listened to from many worthy sources and methods to be learned from successful people who do what you do, you make the final decision as to how and what to do to further your career.

Sometimes that might mean ignoring all the advice, rolling the dice, and taking a chance. You owe it to yourself to do that when against all common sense your body is positively insisting that you try something radical.

I promise you that regardless of what happens you won't fire yourself.

Zealots

The acting profession has its share of fanatics, whether you're talking about a power-tripping director, the acting teacher as ruler of his kingdom, or the stage mother from hell. They're all out there, but I'm glad to report they are outnumbered by others—the director who loves actors and values their opinions, the caring and tuned in acting instructor, and the perfectly well adjusted stage parent who would probably prefer their kid was playing in the park instead of auditioning for a series lead. Avoid the former as best you can and appreciate the day when you work or meet with the latter.

Also be aware that, perish the thought, some actors fall into the zealot category, too. Generally, it's someone who just can't turn the industry off—even for a minute. If you're calling your agent three times per day, sending postcards to the same casting director every week, sitting in a dark theatre watching ten films per week ostensibly for research, overpublicizing yourself with daily trade ads, or insisting on attending every industry function or party you hear about, then you might be a zealot.

Any of these things done in proper moderation is fine, it's even necessary. Doing them obsessively steers you down a potentially dangerous road.

Inside, we usually know when too much is too much. If you don't, ask around, especially to someone whose opinion you value, and you'll figure out what's too much. Our profession attracts people who are driven by their desire to succeed or just work. You have to be a focused person to succeed, but you cannot allow it to be all consuming.

If you find that acting is the only thing you think about twenty-four hours per day, seven days per week, then, yes, you might be a zealot. I'd suggest a nice vacation, therapy, a short-term hiatus, a new hobby, or a really good book (not this one, however) to wean you away from the business. Just do this part of the way anyway, because to achieve staying power in our field, you'll need a work ethic that borders on quasi zealotness. So work hard and do what you need to do, but don't cross that line where the career climb eclipses everything else in your life. Happiness comes when you are able to appreciate where you are right now, and right now isn't a bad place to be.

Zero Auditions

Unhappy actors can almost always be traced back to their recent audition count. You show me a busy auditioner and I'll show you one contented thespian—not as happy as a performer who has an actual job mind you but a pretty satisfied person nonetheless. Conversely, when things slow up, and they eventually do for almost everyone, actors start getting concerned, worried, terrified, or paranoid—not necessarily in that order. The reality is, though, that slowdowns are a common fact of life to the surviving and succeeding actor.

So if a mere slowdown causes all manner of mental anguish, you can only imagine how much anxiety the infamous zilch, zippo, zero audition phase creates—tons and it never gets easier. But that's an unmitigated reality of the acting profession at times—not getting auditions at all. Thankfully, for most professionals, it's something they can survive if they don't let it overcome them first.

Let's assume it's been six or eight weeks with nary a blip on your audition meter. Do you sit back quietly and figure it's just a bad time or are you going to do something to make it stop? If it's the latter, you'll likely come out of your zero phase much more quickly than the next actor. You could get very aggressive to stop the bleeding only to find yourself inactive for yet another month or two. Then again, if it's been three months, you'd likely be more concerned with getting a new agent than the next audition.

As CEO of your own business, you have to get the company moving. You've got to pick up the phone, mail the postcards, push the agent to find opportunities, get new headshots, locate a new teacher, or reedit your demo tape, anything to shake a few leaves off the tree. This isn't a rehearsal folks, it's your career.

It might go against your artist sensibility to start pushing the people who you genuinely like, such as your agent, but you have to do that or else risk them forgetting you altogether. That doesn't just happen to actors who don't book work. An actor who has a hot streak going can almost as easily slip off his agent's radar. Don't allow it to happen. This business is about marketing. If you plan on being discovered by some grand osmosis, that won't happen either. You've got to attack it head on and be relentless.

You didn't deserve this audition stoppage, but it befell you. It wasn't your talent, your fate, or your fault, it was just your turn. All the other actors have that experience, too. It's what you do about it that separates you from the others. The good news is that these phases pass for those who exercise their survival skills.

Then before you know it, you're back out there with sides in your hands. You're auditioning again and before long you zero right in and get the role. Hollywood, there's no place like it.

Concluding Thoughts

Surviving actors are great learners. Because we aren't going to get most of the jobs we want, we learn to come away from each audition as more enlightened actors. The bottom line is that you will not get every part, not even most of them. There are just too many variations and possibilities that get in the way. But you can get your fair share, and maybe even more than that, if you continue to hone, learn, and grow. You could even be the next big thing, but just in case you aren't there yet, listen to the words of those I asked about surviving and succeeding in this business:

> **Manager Phil Brock:** "It's so hard to be a working actor in this business. If you can say you went thirty or forty years as an actor and that was your job, then you have succeeded. The other stuff comes and goes. Fame is fleeting, but if you can say I've made a career of this, you have to be really proud of that."

> **Acting Teacher Daphne Eckler Kirby:** "I think you have to have a very warm and engaging and confident personality. You have to be generous of spirit so the people that you're working with, from agents to producers to casting directors, really feel appreciated by you."

> **Commercial Caster Robert Ferret:** "You grow. We went to a show the other night and there was an actor performing we had seen twice before, but this night he was just stellar. You can tell he had gotten into where he was supposed to be, everything had come to a realization for him and he'd just moved himself up to the next level. Now he'll be coming in for us even more."

> **Casting Director Jeff Gerrard:** "Approach your work naturally and honestly. Listen to your fellow actor. That's what acting is all about. It's listening, it's reacting, it's being in the moment. Those are the people that succeed in the business."

> **Casting Director Brian Myers:** "I get excited when somebody comes in and does something unexpected that is still appropriate to the role or does a very smart read where they have interpreted the material and brought more to it than what's on the page."

> **Casting Director Richard Hicks:** "There are so many things you can't control in the industry. As a non-famous actor you have power almost none of the time. You do have it in that moment when

you're auditioning. So make a pact with yourself not to waste those opportunities."

Agent Kurt Patino: "Actors must show how unique they are in every audition situation. They need to always, always, always keep their energy up, no matter what kind of day they had. They need to bring something special to a character which sets them apart from the pack, not in an extreme or inappropriate way, but in a subtle way that draws an audience to them, be it for one line or a lead role. Have no fear!"

Casting Director Lisa Miller Katz: "I think it's important to have the ability to audition well, feel good about your choices and then walk out of the room and put it away and literally not think about it again. . . . You have to compartmentalize this stuff, put it in a box and just not go back there. If you get it, great, fantastic. If not, it's good-bye to that. Say to yourself, 'I was really good in that audition, I did a good job and what am I going to have for dinner.'"

Actor Oscar Torres: "If you're talented and you're a hard worker and you stay focused and if your goal is to be a working actor, to work, not be a star you're going to be successful. If this is really what you want to do and there's nothing else that you'd rather do, you'll be successful and by the time you're done you've had a very nice career."

Agent Craig Wyckoff: "The determined actor succeeds. It's a lifetime commitment. When I hear an actor say, 'I'm going to give it five or ten years,' I say, then you know what, quit now. Unless you can say there is nothing else you'd be happy doing and you want to do this your entire life, and even if you haven't made it in fifty years from now, you don't care, you'll still be trying, that's when you stay in the industry."

One final thought: I was recently reminded of something; for a business that has such a reputation of being based on chance and what ifs, it's clear to me yet again that you often get out of this field just what you put into it. You can't fully control your destiny as an actor, but you can certainly help to steer it in the right direction. Sure you could get discovered walking across the street on Lankershim, but your chances increase dramatically if you're walking across that very street for an audition on the Universal Lot. You would have gotten there because of all your efforts—training, marketing, finding an agent or manager, and being a professional. There is some chance and randomness to consider in our industry, but the question is, what have you got to go along with that? Nearly every section in this book discusses survival strategies to compete in this city and in our field. The core issue comes down to working hard and giving it your absolute best. It's the only way I've ever known, and I've seen it work.